POCKET GUIDE FOR INTERNATIONAL DIETETICS & NUTRITION TERMINOLOGY (IDNT) REFERENCE MANUAL:

Standardized Language for the Nutrition Care Process

Fourth Edition

D1222332

Pocket Guide for INTERNATIONAL DIETETICS &
NUTRITION TERMINOLOGY (IDNT) REFERENCE MANUAL:
Standardized Language for the Nutrition Care Process
Fourth Edition

ISBN: 978-0-88091-468-0

Academy of Nutrition and Dietetics
120 South Riverside Plaza
Suite 2000
Chicago, IL 60606-6995
800/877-1600
www.eatright.org

The views expressed in this publication are those of the authors and do not necessarily reflect policies and/or official positions of the Academy of Nutrition and Dietetics. Mention of product names in this publication does not constitute endorsement by the authors or the Academy of Nutrition and Dietetics. The Academy of Nutrition and Dietetics disclaims responsibility for the application of the information contained herein.

10 9 8 7 6 5 4 3 2 1

Table of Contents

ASSESSMENT

DIAGNOSIS

INTERVENTION

MONITOR & EVAL

Suggested references for each step are available in the *International Dietetics and Nutrition Terminology (IDNT) Reference Manual*, Fourth Edition. Several additional resources are available on the Academy's website (www.eatright.org). Sign in as a member and select Nutrition Care Process from the sidebar.

4th Edition

Nutrition Care Process Summary

Introduction

Continually emerging from the Academy of Nutrition and Dietetics' strategic plan are priority actions that guide committees, workgroups, and taskforces in creating tools to advance the dietetics profession. In 2002, to achieve the Academy's strategic goals of promoting the demand for food and nutrition professionals and to help such professionals be more competitive in the marketplace, the Academy Quality Management Committee appointed the Nutrition Care Model Workgroup. This Workgroup developed the Nutrition Care Process and Model, a systematic process describing how food and nutrition professionals provide care to patients/clients (1).

The Nutrition Care Process (NCP) is designed to improve the consistency and quality of individualized care for patients/clients or groups and the predictability of the patient/client outcomes. It is not intended to standardize nutrition care for each patient/client, but to establish a standardized process for providing care.

> **Special Note:** The terms **patient(s)/client(s)** are used in association with the NCP; however, the process is also intended for use with groups. In addition, family members or caregivers are an essential asset to the patient/client and food and nutrition professional in the NCP. Therefore, **groups, populations, families, and caregivers** of patients/clients are implied each time a reference is made to patient/client.

There are four steps in the process:
- Nutrition assessment
- Nutrition diagnosis
- Nutrition intervention
- Nutrition monitoring and evaluation

Three of the NCP steps are very familiar to food and nutrition professionals, and nutrition textbooks skillfully cover their content—nutrition assessment, nutrition intervention, and nutrition monitoring and evaluation. However, the Workgroup identified a less well defined aspect of nutrition care: nutrition diagnosis. Further, it recognized that a standard taxonomy for the second step in the process would greatly enhance the profession's ability to document, communicate, and research the impact of nutrition care.

As a result, the Academy's Nutrition Care Process/Standardized Language (NCP/SL) Committee was formed to create a taxonomy for the profession's unique nutrition diagnosis language. The language was described during presentations at the 2005 Food and Nutrition Conference and Exhibition and made available in a publication at that meeting (2). The nutrition diagnosis language is undergoing study in a number of research projects. Future modifications to the language will be made based on research results.

The NCP/SL Committee has examined in-depth all four NCP steps and published a standardized language for nutrition assessment, nutrition diagnosis, nutrition intervention, and nutrition monitoring and evaluation.

Nutrition Care Process Steps

Step 1: Nutrition Assessment

Nutrition assessment is a systematic method for obtaining, verifying, and interpreting data needed to identify nutrition-related problems, their causes, and their significance. It is an ongoing, nonlinear, dynamic process that involves initial data collection, but also continual reassessment and analysis of the patient/client's status compared to specified criteria. From the nutrition assessment data, the food and nutrition professional is able to determine whether a nutrition diagnosis/problem exists. This step, while well known to food and nutrition professionals, will be enhanced by the use of standardized nutrition assessment language for communicating about patients/clients with similar problems.

The nutrition assessment terms are identified and grouped into five domains:
- Food/Nutrition-Related History
- Anthropometric Measurements
- Biochemical Data, Medical Tests, and Procedures
- Nutrition-Focused Physical Findings
- Client History

Nutrition assessment begins after a patient/client referral or as a result of positive nutrition screening, when it is determined that the patient/client may benefit from nutrition care. Nutrition assessment leads to the appropriate determination of whether a nutrition diagnosis/problem exists. If so, the food and nutrition professional correctly diagnoses the problem and creates a PES (Problem, Etiology, Signs/Symptoms) statement in Step 2 of the NCP. In addition, food and nutrition professionals develop the plan for continuation of care or convey the need for further information or testing. If upon the completion of an initial assessment or reassessment it is determined that a nutrition problem does not exist or cannot be modified by further nutrition care, discharge or discontinuation from the episode of nutrition care may be appropriate (3).

Standardized language facilitates more effective comparison of nutrition assessment findings. To this end, the NCP/SL Committee has described the standardized language, data collection, and evaluation approach for nutrition assessment. Many opportunities for research exist in nutrition assessment, which will help determine the most appropriate nutrition assessment data to use for individuals and populations in various practice settings.

Step 2: Nutrition Diagnosis

Nutrition diagnosis is a critical step between nutrition assessment and nutrition intervention. The purpose of a standardized nutrition diagnosis language is to describe nutrition problems consistently so that they are clear within and outside the profession. The standardized language enhances communication and documentation of nutrition care, and it provides a minimum data set and common data elements for future research.

In simple terms, a food and nutrition professional identifies and labels a specific nutrition diagnosis (problem) that, in general, he or she is responsible for treating independently (e.g., excessive carbohydrate intake). With nutrition intervention, the nutrition diagnosis ideally resolves, or at least the signs and symptoms improve. In contrast, a medical diagnosis describes a disease or pathology of organs or body systems (e.g., diabetes). In some instances, such as the nutrition diagnosis Swallowing difficulty (NC-1.1), food and nutrition professionals are labeling or diagnosing the functional problem that has a nutritional consequence. Food and nutrition professionals do not identify medical diagnoses; they diagnose phenomena in the nutrition domain.

Academy's NCP/SL Committee developed a framework that outlines three domains within which the nutrition diagnoses/problems fall:

- Intake
- Clinical
- Behavioral-Environmental

Reference sheets were developed to describe each nutrition diagnosis and incorporate expert input and research feedback.

No nutrition diagnosis at this time (NO-1.1) may be documented if the assessment indicates that no nutrition problem currently exists that warrants a nutrition intervention.

This step in the Nutrition Care Process results in the documentation of the nutrition diagnosis (PES) statement. This statement is composed of three distinct components: the problem (P), the etiology (E) and the signs and symptoms (S). The PES statement is derived from the clustering and synthesis of information gathered during nutrition assessment.

Essential to the understanding of the nutrition problem is the identification of the etiology, or cause or contributing risk factor, of the problem. The Committee has defined the categories of etiologies so practitioners and researchers can better understand the etiology concept and intent, which leads to the most likely nutrition intervention. The Nutrition Diagnosis Etiology Matrix is available on the Academy's website and in the online IDNT Reference Manual.

Step 3: Nutrition Intervention

Nutrition intervention is the third step in the Nutrition Care Process. Nutrition interventions are specific actions used to remedy a nutrition diagnosis/problem, and can be used with individuals, groups, or the community at large. These nutrition interventions are intended to change a nutrition-related behavior, environmental condition, or aspect of nutritional health. A food and nutrition professional collaborates, whenever possible, with the patient/client(s) and other health care providers during the nutrition intervention.

Nutrition intervention consists of two interrelated components—planning and implementation. Planning involves prioritizing the nutrition diagnoses; conferring with the patient and others; consulting practice guides and policies; jointly establishing goals; and defining the nutrition prescription and identifying specific nutrition intervention(s). Implementing the nutrition intervention is the action phase, which includes carrying out and communicating the plan of care, continuing the data collection, and revising the nutrition intervention, as warranted, based on the patient/client response. This step cannot be completed unless both components are in place to support the nutrition intervention.

The nutrition intervention is almost always aimed at the etiology (E) of the nutrition diagnosis/problem identified in the PES statement. In very specific instances, the nutrition intervention is directed at reducing/eliminating the effects of the signs and symptoms (S). Generally, the signs and symptoms form the basis for the next step in the Nutrition Care Process: nutrition monitoring and evaluation (Step 4).

Four domains of nutrition intervention have been identified:
- Food and/or Nutrient Delivery
- Nutrition Education
- Nutrition Counseling
- Coordination of Nutrition Care

The terminology is defined and reference sheets for each specific nutrition intervention are available for use. It is believed that the information necessary for medical record documentation, billing, and the description of the nutrition interventions for research are included in the terminology.

A food and nutrition professional will note that while some interventions are closely related (e.g., education and counseling), the terms are intentionally separated to distinguish between them. Additionally, specific descriptors of a nutrition intervention encounter (i.e., interactions, visits, contacts, sessions) are provided to assist a food and nutrition professional with the details of his or her encounters with the patient/client(s). Examples of descriptors include encounters with individuals or groups, face-to-face or electronically conducted encounters, and the degree to which the food and nutrition professional is responsible for the patient/client care.

Step 4: Nutrition Monitoring and Evaluation

The purpose of nutrition monitoring and evaluation is to quantify progress made by the patient/client in meeting nutrition care goals. During the monitoring and evaluation process, nutrition care outcomes—the desired results of nutrition care—have been defined, and specific indicators that can be measured and compared to established criteria have been identified. Nutrition monitoring and evaluation tracks patient/client outcomes relevant to the nutrition diagnosis and intervention plans and goals.

Selection of appropriate nutrition care indicators is determined by the nutrition diagnosis and its etiology, the signs or symptoms, and the nutrition intervention used. The medical diagnosis and health care outcome goals and quality management goals for nutrition also influence the nutrition care indicators that are chosen. Other factors, such as practice setting, patient/client population, and disease state and/or severity, affect indicator selection.

The nutrition monitoring and evaluation terms are combined with the nutrition assessment terms and organized in four domains:

- Food/Nutrition-Related History
- Anthropometric Measurements
- Biochemical Data, Medical Tests, and Procedures
- Nutrition-Focused Physical Findings

There are no nutrition care outcomes associated with the domain entitled Client History; items from this domain are used for nutrition assessment only and do not change as a result of nutrition intervention.

During this step, food and nutrition professionals monitor the patient/client progress by determining whether the nutrition intervention is being implemented and by providing evidence that the nutrition intervention is or is not changing the patient/client behavior or nutritional/health status. Food and nutrition professionals measure outcomes by selecting the appropriate nutrition care indicator(s) and comparing the findings with nutrition prescription/intervention goals, and/or reference standards. The use of standardized indicators and criteria increases the validity and reliability of the outcome data and facilitates electronic charting, coding, and outcomes measurement.

Implementation of the Nutrition Care Process and Future Directions

Publications and Resources

Food and nutrition professionals are implementing the Nutrition Care Process. This new *International Dietetics and Nutrition Terminology (IDNT) Reference Manual* provides extensive detail and explanation about the complete standardized language for dietetics.

Toolkits are available to support Nutrition Care Process implementation and continuing education. For more information, please see the Bibliography and Resources section of this manual or the Academy website (www.eatright.org) in the Nutrition Care Process section.

Toolkits are also available from the Academy for the online Evidence-Based Nutrition Practice Guidelines, which are based on evidence analyses. They contain sample forms and examples incorporating standardized language terms in the Nutrition Care Process steps. These are available for purchase from the Academy at the Store tab of the Academy Evidence Analysis Library (www.andevidencelibrary.com). Food and nutrition professionals may also find useful the extensive resources, including patient/client case studies, a performance improvement case, audit tools and downloadable presentations, provided on the Academy website in the Nutrition Care Process section.

Members have completed numerous presentations and newsletter articles for national, state, and Dietetic Practice Group audiences. The Academy also facilitates the Peer Network for the Nutrition Care Process (PNNCP), a network of food and nutrition professionals who have led the way in implementing the Nutrition Care Process in their facilities and communities. A contact list for members of the PNNCP is available on the Academy's website.

Billing for Nutrition Encounters

As appropriate to the situation and payer, registered dietitians (RDs) may bill for services they provide during encounters with patients/clients, including but not limited to medical nutrition therapy (MNT) (defined at www.eatright.org/scope > Definition of terms). Many third-party payers, such as the Centers for Medicare and Medicaid Services, require use of the MNT Current Procedural Terminology (CPT) codes on claims submitted for MNT services provided by RDs.

MNT CPT Code Descriptors

97802 Medical nutrition therapy; initial assessment and intervention, individual, face-to-face with the patient, each 15 minutes
97803 Reassessment and intervention, individual, face-to-face with the patient, each 15 minutes
97804 Group (2 or more individual[s]), each 30 minutes
CPT codes, descriptions, and material only are copyright 2012 American Medical Association. All Rights Reserved. CPT is a registered trademark of the American Medical Association.

Compared with other CPT codes, the MNT CPT codes best describe services that food and nutrition professionals and RDs provide to patients/clients receiving medical nutrition therapy for a particular chronic disease or condition. The MNT CPT codes are time-based codes—15-minute and 30-minute increments of time for individual or group MNT, respectively. RDs typically report multiple units of the MNT CPT code on claims for initial, follow-up, and group MNT visits. The total number of units of the MNT code reported for one encounter is determined by the time spent interacting (face-to-face) with the patient/client. In addition, RDs normally provide MNT and other nutrition services over several encounters with the patient/client, based on nutrition practice guidelines, patient/client needs, interests and medical necessity. Multiple visits are needed to help the patient/client achieve goals, desired behavior changes, and/or expected outcomes.

RDs may use other CPT codes when providing nutrition education and training and other nutrition and nutrition-related services. Check payer policies to determine covered services and codes that can be used on claims. For additional detailed coding, coverage, and Medicare MNT resources, refer to the Academy website (www.eatright.org) in the Coding, Coverage, and Compliance or Medicare MNT sections.

International Information Sharing and Standardized Medical Languages

In 2005, the American Dietetic Association (ADA; now the Academy) Foundation funded an ADA-hosted meeting to expand the dialogue with other international dietetic associations about the ADA's standardized nutrition diagnosis language and similar efforts by other associations. The meeting also initiated a dialogue among the foremost medical informatics organizations and the international nutrition and dietetics community. As a result of this dialogue:

- The ADA hosted an international meeting in September 2010 for international dietetic associations and groups to share efforts and questions on implementation of the NCP and the IDNT or other standardized processes and languages. Representatives present included members of the International Confederation of Dietetic Associations, American Overseas Dietetic Association, British Dietetic Association, Dietetic Association of Australia, Dietitians of Canada, Hungarian Dietetic Association, Israel Dietetic Association, Associacao Brasileira de Nutricao - ASBRAN (Brazil), Kenya Bureau of Standards (KEBS), Malaysia Dietetic Association, Turkish Dietetic Association, Dutch Dietetic Association, Swedish Association of Clinical Dietitians, and a representative from Mexico.

- International Confederation of Dietetics Associations received updates on Nutrition Care Process (NCP) and International Dietetics and Nutrition Terminology (IDNT) activities and distributed information to international dietetic associations about translation and publication rights for the IDNT and recruitment of international expert reviewers for the Fourth Edition of IDNT.

- A presentation regarding the NCP was presented at the XV International Congress of Dietetics on September 8–11, 2008 in Yokohama, Japan.

- The Dietitians Association of Australia has initiated a research study evaluating the face validity of the nutrition diagnoses.

- The Dutch Dietetic Association (Nederlandse Vereniging van Diëtisten) has requested permission to use the nutrition diagnoses in their health care databases.

- The Japanese Dietetic Association and the South Korean Dietetic Association have agreements to translate the *IDNT Reference Manual*.

- Dietitians of Canada has published a summary paper in English and French describing the NCP. Work is underway for a French translation of the IDNT in 2012.

- The Association of Clinical Dietitians in Sweden made the NCP a focus of their 2011 annual meeting with a debut of a Swedish translation of the IDNT and terms and definitions.

- The Association of Dietitians of Israel is exploring the potential adoption of both the NCP and IDNT in the national health system. Two presentations and a workshop have already taken place.

Indeed, as the world moves fully into electronic health care records, health informatics, and common databases, the international community of nutrition and food and nutrition professionals has the opportunity to work in partnership with the medical informatics organizations to ensure that data elements critical to capturing nutrition care are included in databases and collected in a consistent way.

Summary

From conception of the Nutrition Care Process in 2002 through its implementation now, the NCP/SL Committee continues to update the Academy's House of Delegates, the Board of Directors, and members through reports, articles, case studies, presentations, publications, and the Academy website.

However, to see the strategic goals of an increased demand for food and nutrition professionals who are more competitive in the marketplace come to fruition, practitioners need to take a historic step by implementing the Nutrition Care Process today.

References

1. Writing Group of the Nutrition Care Process/Standardized Language Committee. Nutrition Care Process and Model part I: The 2008 update. *J Am Diet Assoc*. 2008;108:1113-1117.

2. American Dietetic Association. *Nutrition Diagnosis: A Critical Step in the Nutrition Care Process*. Chicago, IL: American Dietetic Association; 2006.

3. Writing Group of the Nutrition Care Process/Standardized Language Committee. Nutrition Care Process part II: Using the International Dietetics and Nutrition Terminology to document the nutrition care process. *J Am Diet Assoc*. 2008;108:1287-1293.

4. Academy of Nutrition and Dietetics. Evidence-based Toolkits. Available at: www.andevidencelibrary.com/store. Accessed January 26, 2012.

SNAPshot
NCP Step 1: Nutrition Assessment

What is the purpose of nutrition assessment? The purpose is to obtain, verify, and interpret data needed to identify nutrition-related problems, their causes, and significance. It is an ongoing, nonlinear, dynamic process that involves initial data collection, but also continual reassessment and analysis of the patient/client's status compared to specified criteria. This contrasts with nutrition monitoring and evaluation data where food and nutrition professionals use similar, or even the same, data to determine changes in patient/client* behavior or nutritional status and the efficacy of nutrition intervention.

How does a food and nutrition professional determine where to obtain nutrition assessment data? It depends on the practice setting. For individuals, data can come directly from the patient/client through interview, observation and measurements, a medical record, and the referring health care provider. For population groups, data from surveys, administrative data sets, and epidemiological or research studies are used. A nutrition assessment matrix that links nutrition assessment parameters with nutrition diagnoses is available to assist practitioners in identifying nutrition diagnoses.

How are Nutrition Assessment data organized? In five categories:

> **Food/Nutrition-Related History**—*Food and nutrient intake, food and nutrient administration, medication/herbal supplement use, knowledge/beliefs, food and supplies availability, physical activity, nutrition quality of life*
>
> **Anthropometric Measurements**—*Height, weight, body mass index (BMI), growth pattern indices/percentile ranks, and weight history*
>
> **Biochemical Data, Medical Tests, and Procedures**—*Lab data (e.g., electrolytes, glucose) and tests (e.g., gastric emptying time, resting metabolic rate)*
>
> **Nutrition-Focused Physical Findings**—*Physical appearance, muscle and fat wasting, swallow function, appetite, and affect*
>
> **Client History**—*Personal history, medical/health/family history, treatments and complementary/alternative medicine use, and social history*

What is done with the nutrition assessment data? Nutrition assessment data (indicators) are compared to criteria, relevant norms and standards, for interpretation and decision making. These may be national, institutional, or regulatory norms and standards. Nutrition assessment findings are documented in nutrition diagnosis statements and nutrition intervention goal setting.

Patient/client refers to individuals, groups, populations, family members, and/or caregivers.

Critical thinking during this step...
- Determining appropriate data to collect
- Determining the need for additional information
- Selecting assessment tools and procedures that match the situation
- Applying assessment tools in valid and reliable ways
- Distinguishing relevant from irrelevant data
- Distinguishing important from unimportant data
- Validating the data

Is there a standardized language or taxonomy for nutrition assessment? Yes. A standard taxonomy for nutrition assessment supports a consistent approach to the NCP and enhances communication and research. The terms for nutrition assessment and nutrition monitoring and evaluation are combined, because the data points are the same or related; however, the data purpose and use are distinct in these two steps.

Are food and nutrition professionals limited to the nutrition assessment data included in the matrix and used in the nutrition diagnoses? Nutrition assessment data listed in the nutrition diagnoses reference sheets are undergoing study and research to confirm (validate) which data are most relevant to specific nutrition diagnoses. However, proposals for additions or revisions can be submitted using the Procedure for Nutrition Controlled Vocabulary/Terminology Maintenance/Review available from the Academy.

Detailed information about this step can be found in the Academy of Nutrition and Dietetics' International Dietetics and Nutrition Terminology (IDNT) Reference Manual: Standardized Language for the Nutrition Care Process, Fourth Edition.

Nutrition Assessment and Monitoring and Evaluation Terminology

This is a combined list of Nutrition Assessment and Monitoring and Evaluation terms. Indicators that are shaded are used ONLY for nutrition assessment. The rest of the indicators are used for assessment and monitoring and evaluation. Each term has an Academy unique identifier, a five-digit number (e.g., 99999) following the alpha-numeric IDNT code. Neither should be visible in nutrition documentation. The Academy unique identifier is for data tracking purposes in electronic health records.

FOOD/NUTRITION-RELATED HISTORY (FH)

Food and nutrient intake, food and nutrient administration, medication and complementary/alternative medicine use, knowledge/beliefs/attitudes, behavior, food and supply availability, physical activity and function, nutrition-related patient/client-centered measures.

Food and Nutrient Intake (1)

Composition and adequacy of food and nutrient intake, meal and snack patterns, current and previous diets and/or food modifications, and eating environment.

Energy Intake (1.1)

Total energy intake from all sources including food, beverages, breastmilk/formula, supplements, and via enteral and parenteral routes.

Energy intake (1.1.1)
❑ Total energy intake	FH-1.1.1.1	10005

Food and Beverage Intake (1.2)

Type, amount, and pattern of intake of foods and food groups, indices of diet quality, intake of fluids, breastmilk and infant formula

Fluid/beverage intake (1.2.1)
❑ Oral fluids	FH-1.2.1.1	10008
❑ Food-derived fluids	FH-1.2.1.2	10009
❑ Liquid meal replacement or supplement	FH-1.2.1.3	10010

Food intake (1.2.2)
❑ Amount of food	FH-1.2.2.1	10012
❑ Types of food/meals	FH-1.2.2.2	10013
❑ Meal/snack pattern	FH-1.2.2.3	10014
❑ Diet quality index	FH-1.2.2.4	10015
❑ Food variety	FH-1.2.2.5	10016

Breastmilk/infant formula intake (1.2.3)
❑ Breastmilk intake	FH-1.2.3.1	10018
❑ Infant formula intake	FH-1.2.3.2	10019

Enteral and Parenteral Nutrition Intake (1.3)

Specialized nutrition support intake from all sources, e.g., enteral and parenteral routes.

Enteral nutrition intake (1.3.1)
❑ Formula/solution	FH-1.3.1.1	10022
❑ Feeding tube flush	FH-1.3.1.2	10023

Parenteral nutrition intake (1.3.2)
❑ Formula/solution	FH-1.3.2.1	10025
❑ IV fluids	FH-1.3.2.2	10026

Bioactive Substance Intake (1.4)

Alcohol, plant stanol and sterol esters, soy protein, psyllium and β-glucan, and caffeine intake from all sources, e.g., food, beverages, supplements, and via enteral and parenteral routes.

Alcohol intake (1.4.1)
❑ Drink size/volume	FH-1.4.1.1	10029
❑ Frequency	FH-1.4.1.2	10030
❑ Pattern of alcohol consumption	FH-1.4.1.3	10031

Bioactive substance intake (1.4.2)
❑ Plant stanol esters	FH-1.4.2.1	10034
❑ Plant sterol esters	FH-1.4.2.2	10807
❑ Soy protein	FH-1.4.2.3	10035
❑ Psyllium	FH-1.4.2.4	10827
❑ β-glucan	FH-1.4.2.5	10037
❑ Food additives (*specify*)	FH-1.4.2.6	10038
❑ Other (*specify*)	FH-1.4.2.7	10039

Caffeine intake (1.4.3)
❑ Total caffeine	FH-1.4.3.1	10041

Macronutrient Intake (1.5)

Fat and cholesterol, protein, carbohydrate, and fiber intake from all sources including food, beverages, supplements, and via enteral and parenteral routes.

Fat and cholesterol intake (1.5.1)
❑ Total fat	FH-1.5.1.1	10044
❑ Saturated fat	FH-1.5.1.2	10045
❑ Trans fatty acids	FH-1.5.1.3	10046
❑ Polyunsaturated fat	FH-1.5.1.4	10047
❑ Monounsaturated fat	FH-1.5.1.5	10048
❑ Omega-3 fatty acids	FH-1.5.1.6	10049
❑ Dietary cholesterol	FH-1.5.1.7	10050
❑ Essential fatty acids	FH-1.5.1.8	10051

Protein intake (1.5.2)
❑ Total protein	FH-1.5.2.1	10053
❑ High biological value protein	FH-1.5.2.2	10054
❑ Casein	FH-1.5.2.3	10055
❑ Whey	FH-1.5.2.4	10056
❑ Amino acids	FH-1.5.2.5	10057
❑ Essential amino acids	FH-1.5.2.6	10058

Carbohydrate intake (1.5.3)
❑ Total carbohydrate	FH-1.5.3.1	10060
❑ Sugar	FH-1.5.3.2	10061
❑ Starch	FH-1.5.3.3	10062
❑ Glycemic index	FH-1.5.3.4	10063
❑ Glycemic load	FH-1.5.3.5	10064
❑ Source of carbohydrate	FH-1.5.3.6	10065

| ❑ Insulin-to-carbohydrate ratio | FH-1.5.3.7 | 10066 |

Fiber intake (1.5.4)

❑ Total fiber	FH-1.5.4.1	10068
❑ Soluble fiber	FH-1.5.4.2	10069
❑ Insoluble fiber	FH-1.5.4.3	10070

Micronutrient Intake (1.6)

Vitamin and mineral intake from all sources, e.g., food, beverages, supplements, and via enteral and parenteral routes.

Vitamin intake (1.6.1)

❑ A (1)		10073
❑ C (2)		10074
❑ D (3)		10075
❑ E (4)		10076
❑ K (5)		10077
❑ Thiamin (6)		10078
❑ Riboflavin (7)		10079
❑ Niacin (8)		10080
❑ Folate (9)		10081
❑ B6 (10)		10082
❑ B12 (11)		10083
❑ Pantothenic acid (12)		10084
❑ Biotin (13)		10085
❑ Multivitamin (14)		10086

Mineral/element intake (1.6.2)

❑ Calcium (1)		10089
❑ Chloride (2)		10090
❑ Iron (3)		10091
❑ Magnesium (4)		10092
❑ Potassium (5)		10093
❑ Phosphorus (6)		10094
❑ Sodium (7)		10095
❑ Zinc (8)		10096
❑ Sulfate (9)		10097
❑ Fluoride (10)		10098
❑ Copper (11)		10099
❑ Iodine (12)		10100
❑ Selenium (13)		10101
❑ Manganese (14)		10102
❑ Chromium (15)		10103
❑ Molybdenum (16)		10104
❑ Boron (17)		10105
❑ Cobalt (18)		10106
❑ Multi-mineral (19)		10107
❑ Multi-trace element (20)		10108

Food and Nutrient Administration (2)

Current and previous diets and/or food modifications, eating environment, and enteral and parenteral nutrition administration.

Diet History (2.1)

Description of food and drink regularly provided or consumed, past diets followed or prescribed and counseling received, and the eating environment.

Diet order (2.1.1)

❑ General, healthful diet	FH-2.1.1.1	10113
❑ Modified diet	FH-2.1.1.2	10114
❑ Enteral nutrition order	FH-2.1.1.3	10115
❑ Parenteral nutrition order	FH-2.1.1.4	10116

Diet experience (2.1.2)

❑ Previously prescribed diets	FH-2.1.2.1	10118
❑ Previous diet/nutrition education/counseling	FH-2.1.2.2	10119
❑ Self-selected diet/s followed	FH-2.1.2.3	10120
❑ Dieting attempts	FH-2.1.2.4	10121
❑ Food allergies	FH-2.1.2.5	10805
❑ Food intolerance	FH-2.1.2.6	10806

Eating environment (2.1.3)

❑ Location	FH-2.1.3.1	10123
❑ Atmosphere	FH-2.1.3.2	10124
❑ Caregiver/companion	FH-2.1.3.3	10125
❑ Appropriate breastfeeding accommodations/facility	FH-2.1.3.4	10126
❑ Eats alone	FH-2.1.3.5	10127

Enteral and parenteral nutrition administration (2.1.4)

❑ Enteral access	FH-2.1.4.1	10129
❑ Parenteral access	FH-2.1.4.2	10130
❑ Body position, EN	FH-2.1.4.3	10804

Medication and Complementary/ Alternative Medicine Use (3)

Prescription and over-the-counter medications, including herbal preparations and complementary/ alternative medicine products used.

Medications (3.1)

❑ Prescription medication use	FH-3.1.1	10820
❑ OTC medication use	FH-3.1.2	10134
❑ Misuse of medication	FH-3.1.3	10135

Complementary/Alternative Medicine (3.2)

| ❑ Nutrtion-related complementary/alternative medicine use | FH-3.2.1 | 10137 |

Knowledge/Beliefs/Attitudes (4)

Understanding of nutrition-related concepts and conviction of the truth and feelings/emotions toward some nutrition-related statement or phenomenon, along with readiness to change nutrition-related behaviors.

Food and nutrition knowledge/skill (4.1)

| ❑ Area(s) and level of knowledge/skill | FH-4.1.1 | 10848 |
| ❑ Diagnosis specific or global nutrition-related knowledge score | FH-4.1.2 | 10143 |

Beliefs and attitudes (4.2)

❑ Conflict with personal/ family value system	FH-4.2.1	10145
❑ Distorted body image	FH-4.2.2	10146
❑ End-of-life decisions	FH-4.2.3	10147
❑ Motivation	FH-4.2.4	10148
❑ Preoccupation with food/nutrients	FH-4.2.5	10149

❏ Preoccupation with weight	FH-4.2.6	10150
❏ Readiness to change nutrition-related behaviors	FH-4.2.7	10151
❏ Self-efficacy	FH-4.2.8	10152
❏ Self-talk/cognitions	FH-4.2.9	10153
❏ Unrealistic nutrition-related goals	FH-4.2.10	10154
❏ Unscientific beliefs/attitudes	FH-4.2.11	10155
❏ Food preferences	FH-4.2.12	10156
❏ Emotions	FH-4.2.13	10157

Behavior (5)

Patient/client activities and actions, which influence achievement of nutrition-related goals.

Adherence (5.1)

❏ Self-reported adherence score	FH-5.1.1	10160
❏ Nutrition visit attendance	FH-5.1.2	10161
❏ Ability to recall nutrition goals	FH-5.1.3	10162
❏ Self-monitoring at agreed upon rate	FH-5.1.4	10163
❏ Self-management as agreed upon	FH-5.1.5	10164

Avoidance behavior (5.2)

❏ Avoidance	FH-5.2.1	10166
❏ Restrictive eating	FH-5.2.2	10167
❏ Cause of avoidance behavior	FH-5.2.3	10168

Bingeing and purging behavior (5.3)

| ❏ Binge eating behavior | FH-5.3.1 | 10170 |
| ❏ Purging behavior | FH-5.3.2 | 10171 |

Mealtime behavior (5.4)

❏ Meal duration	FH-5.4.1	10173
❏ Percent of meal time spent eating	FH-5.4.2	10174
❏ Preference to drink rather than eat	FH-5.4.3	10175
❏ Refusal to eat/chew	FH-5.4.4	10176
❏ Spitting food out	FH-5.4.5	10177
❏ Rumination	FH-5.4.6	10178
❏ Patient/client/caregiver fatigue during feeding process resulting in inadequate intake	FH-5.4.7	10179
❏ Willingness to try new foods	FH-5.4.8	10180
❏ Limited number of accepted foods	FH-5.4.9	10181
❏ Rigid sensory preferences	FH-5.4.10	10182

Social network (5.5)

| ❏ Ability to build and utilize social network | FH-5.5.1 | 10184 |

Factors Affecting Access to Food and Food/Nutrition-Related Supplies (6)

Factors that affect intake and availability of a sufficient quantity of safe, healthful food as well as food/nutrition-related supplies.

Food/nutrition program participation (6.1)

❏ Eligibility for government programs	FH-6.1.1	10187
❏ Participation in government programs	FH-6.1.2	10188
❏ Eligibility for community programs	FH-6.1.3	10189
❏ Participation in community programs	FH-6.1.4	10190

Safe food/meal availability (6.2)

❏ Availability of shopping facilities	FH-6.2.1	10192
❏ Procurement of safe food	FH-6.2.2	10800
❏ Appropriate meal preparation facilities	FH-6.2.3	10194
❏ Availability of safe food storage	FH-6.2.4	10195
❏ Appropriate storage technique	FH-6.2.5	10196
❏ Identification of safe food	FH-6.2.6	10801

Safe water availability (6.3)

| ❏ Availability of potable water | FH-6.3.1 | 10198 |
| ❏ Appropriate water decontamination | FH-6.3.2 | 10199 |

Food and nutrition-related supplies availability (6.4)

❏ Access to food and nutrition-related supplies	FH-6.4.1	10201
❏ Access to assistive eating devices	FH-6.4.2	10202
❏ Access to assistive food preparation devices	FH 6.4.3	10203

Physical Activity and Function (7)

Physical activity, cognitive and physical ability to engage in specific tasks, e.g., breastfeeding, self-feeding.

Breastfeeding (7.1)

❏ Initiation of breastfeeding	FH-7.1.1	10206
❏ Duration of breastfeeding	FH-7.1.2	10207
❏ Exclusive breastfeeding	FH-7.1.3	10208
❏ Breastfeeding problems	FH-7.1.4	10209

Nutrition-related ADLs and IADLs (7.2)

❏ Physical ability to complete tasks for meal preparation	FH-7.2.1	10211
❏ Physical ability to self-feed	FH-7.2.2	10212
❏ Ability to position self in relation to plate	FH-7.2.3	10213
❏ Receives assistance with intake	FH 7.2.4	10214

❑ Ability to use adaptive eating devices — FH 7.2.5 — 10215

❑ Cognitive ability to complete tasks for meal preparation — FH-7.2.6 — 10216

❑ Remembers to eat — FH-7.2.7 — 10139

❑ Recalls eating — FH-7.2.8 — 10218

❑ Mini Mental State Examination Score — FH-7.2.9 — 10219

❑ Nutrition-related activities of daily living (ADL) score — FH-7.2.10 — 10220

❑ Nutrition-related instrumental activities of daily living (IADL) score — FH-7.2.11 — 10221

Physical activity (7.3)

❑ Physical activity history — FH-7.3.1 — 10223

❑ Consistency — FH-7.3.2 — 10224

❑ Frequency — FH-7.3.3 — 10225

❑ Duration — FH-7.3.4 — 10226

❑ Intensity — FH-7.3.5 — 10227

❑ Type of physical activity — FH-7.3.6 — 10228

❑ Strength — FH-7.3.7 — 10229

❑ TV/screen time — FH-7.3.8 — 10230

❑ Other sedentary activity time — FH-7.3.9 — 10231

❑ Involuntary physical movement — FH-7.3.10 — 10232

❑ NEAT — FH-7.3.11 — 10233

Factors affecting access to physical activity (7.4)

❑ Neighborhood safety — FH-7.4.1 — 10822

❑ Walkability of neighborhood — FH-7.4.2 — 10823

❑ Proximity to parks/ green space — FH-7.4.3 — 10824

❑ Access to physical activity facilities/programs — FH-7.4.4 — 10825

Nutrition-Related Patient/Client-Centered Measures (8)

Patient/client's perception of his or her nutrition intervention and its impact on life.

Nutrition quality of life (8.1)

❑ Nutrition quality of life responses — FH-8.1.1 — 10236

ANTHROPOMETRIC MEASUREMENTS (AD)

Height, weight, body mass index (BMI), growth pattern indices/percentile ranks, and weight history.

Body composition/growth/weight history (1.1)

❑ Height/length — AD-1.1.1 — 10239

❑ Weight — AD-1.1.2 — 10240

❑ Frame size — AD-1.1.3 — 10241

❑ Weight change — AD-1.1.4 — 10242

❑ Body mass index — AD-1.1.5 — 10243

❑ Growth pattern indices/ percentile ranks — AD-1.1.6 — 10244

❑ Body compartment estimates — AD-1.1.7 — 10245

BIOCHEMICAL DATA, MEDICAL TESTS AND PROCEDURES (BD)

Laboratory data, (e.g., electrolytes, glucose, and lipid panel) and tests (e.g., gastric emptying time, resting metabolic rate).

Acid-base balance (1.1)

❑ Arterial pH — BD-1.1.1 — 10248

❑ Arterial bicarbonate — BD-1.1.2 — 10249

❑ Partial pressure of carbon dioxide in arterial blood, $PaCO_2$ — BD-1.1.3 — 10250

❑ Partial pressure of oxygen in arterial blood, PaO_2 — BD-1.1.4 — 10251

❑ Venous pH — BD-1.1.5 — 10252

❑ Venous bicarbonate — BD-1.1.6 — 10253

Electrolyte and renal profile (1.2)

❑ BUN — BD-1.2.1 — 10255

❑ Creatinine — BD-1.2.2 — 10256

❑ BUN:creatinine ratio — BD-1.2.3 — 10257

❑ Glomerular filtration rate — BD-1.2.4 — 10258

❑ Sodium — BD-1.2.5 — 10259

❑ Chloride — BD-1.2.6 — 10260

❑ Potassium — BD-1.2.7 — 10261

❑ Magnesium — BD-1.2.8 — 10262

❑ Calcium, serum — BD-1.2.9 — 10263

❑ Calcium, ionized — BD-1.2.10 — 10264

❑ Phosphorus — BD-1.2.11 — 10265

❑ Serum osmolality — BD-1.2.12 — 10266

❑ Parathyroid hormone — BD-1.2.13 — 10267

Essential fatty acid profile (1.3)

❑ Triene:Tetraene ratio — BD-1.3.1 — 10269

Gastrointestinal profile (1.4)

❑ Alkaline phosphatase — BD-1.4.1 — 10271

❑ Alanine aminotransferase, ALT — BD-1.4.2 — 10272

❑ Aspartate aminotransferase, AST — BD-1.4.3 — 10273

❑ Gamma glutamyl transferase, GGT — BD-1.4.4 — 10274

❑ Gastric residual volume — BD-1.4.5 — 10275

❑ Bilirubin, total — BD-1.4.6 — 10276

❑ Ammonia, serum — BD-1.4.7 — 10277

❑ Toxicology report, including alcohol — BD-1.4.8 — 10278

❑ Prothrombin time, PT — BD-1.4.9 — 10279

❑ Partial thromboplastin time, PTT — BD-1.4.10 — 10280

❑ INR (ratio) — BD-1.4.11 — 10281

❑ Fecal fat — BD-1.4.12 — 10282

❑ Amylase — BD-1.4.13 — 10283

❑ Lipase — BD-1.4.14 — 10284

❑ Other digestive enzymes (*specify*) — BD-1.4.15 — 10285

❑ D-xylose — BD-1.4.16 — 10286

❑ Hydrogen breath test — BD-1.4.17 — 10287

❑ Intestinal biopsy — BD-1.4.18 — 10288

❑ Stool culture — BD-1.4.19 — 10289

❑ Gastric emptying time — BD-1.4.20 — 10290

❑ Small bowel transit time — BD-1.4.21 — 10291

| ❑ Abdominal films | BD-1.4.22 | 10292 |
| ❑ Swallow study | BD-1.4.23 | 10293 |

Glucose/endocrine profile (1.5)

❑ Glucose, fasting	BD-1.5.1	10295
❑ Glucose, casual	BD-1.5.2	10296
❑ HgbA1c	BD-1.5.3	10297
❑ Preprandial capillary plasma glucose	BD-1.5.4	10298
❑ Peak postprandial capillary plasma glucose	BD-1.5.5	10299
❑ Glucose tolerance test	BD-1.5.6	10300
❑ Cortisol level	BD-1.5.7	10301
❑ IGF-binding protein	BD-1.5.8	10302
❑ Thyroid function tests (TSH, T4, T3)	BD-1.5.9	10303
❑ Pituitary hormone tests (GH, ACTH, LH, FSH)	BD-1.5.10	10826

Inflammatory profile (1.6)

| ❑ C-reactive protein | BD-1.6.1 | 10305 |

Lipid profile (1.7)

❑ Cholesterol, serum	BD-1.7.1	10307
❑ Cholesterol, HDL	BD-1.7.2	10308
❑ Cholesterol, LDL	BD-1.7.3	10309
❑ Cholesterol, non-HDL	BD-1.7.4	10310
❑ Total cholesterol:HDL cholesterol	BD-1.7.5	10311
❑ LDL:HDL	BD-1.7.6	10312
❑ Triglycerides, serum	BD-1.7.7	10313

Metabolic rate profile (1.8)

| ❑ Resting metabolic rate, measured | BD-1.8.1 | 10315 |
| ❑ Respiratory quotient, measured | BD-1.8.2 | 10316 |

Mineral profile (1.9)

❑ Copper, serum or plasma	BD-1.9.1	10318
❑ Iodine, urinary excretion	BD-1.9.2	10319
❑ Zinc, serum or plasma	BD-1.9.3	10320
❑ Boron, serum or plasma	BD-1.9.4	10841
❑ Chromium, serum or urinary	BD-1.9.5	10842
❑ Fluoride, plasma	BD-1.9.6	10843
❑ Manganese, urinary, blood, plasma	BD-1.9.7	10844
❑ Molybdenum, serum	BD-1.9.8	10845
❑ Selenium, serum or urinary	BD-1.9.9	10846

Nutritional anemia profile (1.10)

❑ Hemoglobin	BD-1.10.1	10323
❑ Hematocrit	BD-1.10.2	10324
❑ Mean corpuscular volume	BD-1.10.3	10325
❑ Red blood cell folate	BD-1.10.4	10326
❑ Red cell distribution width	BD-1.10.5	10327
❑ B12, serum	BD-1.10.6	10328
❑ Methylmalonic acid, serum	BD-1.10.7	10329
❑ Folate, serum	BD-1.10.8	10330
❑ Homocysteine, serum	BD-1.10.9	10331
❑ Ferritin, serum	BD-1.10.10	10332
❑ Iron, serum	BD-1.10.11	10333
❑ Total iron-binding capacity	BD-1.10.12	10334
❑ Transferrin saturation	BD-1.10.13	10335

Protein profile (1.11)

❑ Albumin	BD-1.11.1	10337
❑ Prealbumin	BD-1.11.2	10338
❑ Transferrin	BD-1.11.3	10339
❑ Phenylalanine, plasma	BD-1.11.4	10340
❑ Tyrosine, plasma	BD-1.11.5	10341
❑ Amino acid, other, specify	BD-1.11.6	10342
❑ Antibody level, specify	BD-1.11.7	10343
❑ Carbohydrate-deficient transferrin	BD-1.11.8	10847

Urine profile (1.12)

❑ Urine color	BD-1.12.1	10345
❑ Urine osmolality	BD-1.12.2	10346
❑ Urine specific gravity	BD-1.12.3	10347
❑ Urine test, specify	BD-1.12.4	10348
❑ Urine volume	BD-1.12.5	10349

Vitamin profile (1.13)

❑ Vitamin A, serum or plasma retinol	BD-1.13.1	10351
❑ Vitamin C, plasma or serum	BD-1.13.2	10352
❑ Vitamin D, 25-hydroxy	BD-1.13.3	10353
❑ Vitamin E, plasma alpha-tocopherol	BD-1.13.4	10354
❑ Thiamin, activity coefficient for erythrocyte transketolase activity	BD-1.13.5	10355
❑ Riboflavin, activity coefficient for erythrocyte glutathione reductase activity	BD-1.13.6	10356
❑ Niacin, urinary N'methyl-nicotinamide concentration	BD-1.13.7	10357
❑ Vitamin B6, plasma or serum pyridoxal 5'phosphate concentration	BD-1.13.8	10358
❑ Pantothenic acid, urinary pantothenate excretion, plasma	BD-1.13.9	10850
❑ Biotin, urinary 3-hydroxyisovaleric acid excretion or lympho-cyte propionyl-CoA carboxylase in pregnancy, serum	BD-1.13.10	10851

NUTRITION-FOCUSED PHYSICAL FINDINGS (PD)

Findings from an evaluation of body systems, muscle and subcutaneous fat wasting, oral health, suck/ swallow/breathe ability, appetite, and affect.

Nutrition-focused physical findings (1.1)

| ❑ Overall appearance (*specify*) _____ | PD-1.1.1 | 10362 |
| ❑ Body language (*specify*) _____ | PD-1.1.2 | 10363 |

❏ Cardiovascular-pulmonary (*specify*) _____	PD-1.1.3	10364
❏ Extremities, muscles and bones (*specify*) _____	PD-1.1.4	10365
❏ Digestive system (mouth to rectum) (*specify*) _____	PD-1.1.5	10366
❏ Head and eyes (*specify*) _____	PD-1.1.6	10367
❏ Nerves and cognition (*specify*) _____	PD-1.1.7	10368
❏ Skin (*specify*) _____	PD-1.1.8	10369
❏ Vital signs (*specify*) _____	PD-1.1.9	10370

CLIENT HISTORY (CH)
Current and past information related to personal, medical, family, and social history.

Personal History (1)
General patient/client information such as age, gender, race/ethnicity, language, education, and role in family.

Personal data (1.1)
❏ Age	CH-1.1.1	10374
❏ Gender	CH-1.1.2	10375
❏ Race/Ethnicity	CH-1.1.3	10376
❏ Language	CH-1.1.4	10377
❏ Literacy factors	CH-1.1.5	10378
❏ Education	CH-1.1.6	10379
❏ Role in family	CH-1.1.7	10380
❏ Tobacco use	CH-1.1.8	10381
❏ Physical disability	CH-1.1.9	10382
❏ Mobility	CH-1.1.10	10383

Patient/Client/Family Medical/Health History (2)
Patient/client or family disease states, conditions, and illnesses that may have nutritional impact.

Patient/client OR family nutrition-oriented medical/health history (2.1)
Specify issue(s) and whether it is patient/client history (P) or family history (F)

❏ Patient/client chief nutrition complaint (*specify*) _____	CH-2.1.1	10386 P or F
❏ Cardiovascular (*specify*) _____	CH-2.1.2	10387 P or F
❏ Endocrine/metabolism (*specify*) _____	CH-2.1.3	10388 P or F
❏ Excretory (*specify*) _____	CH-2.1.4	10389 P or F
❏ Gastrointestinal (*specify*) _____	CH-2.1.5	10390 P or F
❏ Gynecological (*specify*) _____	CH-2.1.6	10391 P or F
❏ Hematology/oncology (*specify*) _____	CH-2.1.7	10392 P or F
❏ Immune (e.g., food allergies) (*specify*) _____	CH-2.1.8	10393 P or F
❏ Integumentary (*specify*) _____	CH-2.1.9	10394 P or F
❏ Musculoskeletal (*specify*) _____	CH-2.1.10	10395 P or F
❏ Neurological (*specify*) _____	CH-2.1.11	10396 P or F
❏ Psychological (*specify*) _____	CH-2.1.12	10397 P or F
❏ Respiratory (*specify*) _____	CH-2.1.13	10398 P or F
❏ Other (*specify*) _____	CH-2.1.14	10399 P or F

Treatments/therapy (2.2)
Documented medical or surgical treatments that may impact nutritional status of the patient

❏ Medical treatment/therapy (*specify*) _____	CH-2.2.1	10401
❏ Surgical treatment (*specify*) _____	CH-2.2.2	10402
❏ Palliative/end-of-life care (*specify*) _____	CH-2.2.3	10404

Social History (3)
Patient/client socioeconomic status, housing situation, medical care support and involvement in social groups.

Social history (3.1)
❏ Socioeconomic factors (*specify*) _____	CH-3.1.1	10407
❏ Living/housing situation (*specify*) _____	CH-3.1.2	10408
❏ Domestic issues (*specify*) _____	CH-3.1.3	10409
❏ Social and medical support (*specify*) _____	CH-3.1.4	10410
❏ Geographic location of home (*specify*) _____	CH-3.1.5	10411
❏ Occupation (*specify*) _____	CH-3.1.6	10412
❏ Religion (*specify*) _____	CH-3.1.7	10413
❏ History of recent crisis (*specify*) _____	CH-3.1.8	10414
❏ Daily stress level	CH-3.1.9	10415

COMPARATIVE STANDARDS (CS)

Energy Needs (1)
Estimated energy needs (1.1)
❏ Total energy estimated needs	CS-1.1.1	10419
❏ Method for estimating needs	CS-1.1.2	10420

Macronutrient Needs (2)

Estimated fat needs (2.1)

☐ Total fat estimated needs	CS-2.1.1	10423
☐ Type of fat needed	CS-2.1.2	10424
☐ Method for estimating needs	CS-2.1.3	10425

Estimated protein needs (2.2)

☐ Total protein estimated needs	CS-2.2.1	10427
☐ Type of protein needed	CS-2.2.2	10428
☐ Method for estimating needs	CS-2.2.3	10429

Estimated carbohydrate needs (2.3)

☐ Total carbohydrate estimated needs	CS-2.3.1	10431
☐ Type of carbohydrate needed	CS-2.3.2	10432
☐ Method for estimating needs	CS-2.3.3	10433

Estimated fiber needs (2.4)

☐ Total fiber estimated needs	CS-2.4.1	10435
☐ Type of fiber needed	CS-2.4.2	10436
☐ Method for estimating needs	CS-2.4.3	10437

Fluid Needs (3)

Estimated fluid needs (3.1)

☐ Total fluid estimated needs	CS-3.1.1	10440
☐ Method for estimating needs	CS-3.1.2	10441

Micronutrient Needs (4)

Estimated vitamin needs (4.1)

☐ A (1)	10444
☐ C (2)	10445
☐ D (3)	10446
☐ E (4)	10447
☐ K (5)	10448
☐ Thiamin (6)	10449
☐ Riboflavin (7)	10450
☐ Niacin (8)	10451
☐ Folate (9)	10452
☐ B6 (10)	10453
☐ B12 (11)	10454
☐ Pantothenic acid (12)	10455
☐ Biotin (13)	10456
☐ Method for estimating needs (14)	10458

Estimated mineral needs (4.2)

☐ Calcium (1)	10460
☐ Chloride (2)	10461
☐ Iron (3)	10462
☐ Magnesium (4)	10463
☐ Potassium (5)	10464
☐ Phosphorus (6)	10465
☐ Sodium (7)	10466
☐ Zinc (8)	10467
☐ Sulfate (9)	10469
☐ Fluoride (10)	10470
☐ Copper (11)	10471
☐ Iodine (12)	10473
☐ Selenium (13)	10474
☐ Manganese (14)	10475
☐ Chromium (15)	10476
☐ Molybdenum (16)	10477
☐ Boron (17)	10478
☐ Cobalt (18)	10479
☐ Method for estimating needs (19)	10480

Weight and Growth Recommendation (5)

Recommended body weight/body mass Index/growth (5.1)

☐ Ideal/reference body weight (IBW)	CS-5.1.1	10483
☐ Recommended body mass index (BMI)	CS-5.1.2	10484
☐ Desired growth pattern	CS-5.1.3	10485

Energy Intake (FH-1.1.1)

Definition

Amount of energy intake from all sources, e.g., food, beverages, breastmilk/formula, supplements, and via enteral and parenteral routes

> *Note: Whenever possible, nutrient intake data should be considered in combination with clinical, biochemical, anthropometric information, medical diagnosis, clinical status, and/ or other factors as well as diet to provide a valid assessment of nutritional status based on a totality of the evidence.* (Institute of Medicine. Dietary Reference Intakes: Applications *in Dietary Assessment. Washington, DC: National Academies Press; 2000.)*

Nutrition Assessment and Monitoring and Evaluation

Indicators

Total energy intake (specify, e.g., calories, kcal or kJ/day, calories, kcal or kJ/kg/day)

> *Note: Weight and weight change can be found on the Body Composition/Growth/Weight History reference sheet.*

Examples of the measurement methods or data sources for these indicators: Food intake records, 24-hour recall, 3 to 5 day food diary, food frequency questionnaire, caretaker intake records, menu analysis, intake and output records

Typically used with the following domains of nutrition interventions: Food and/or nutrient delivery, nutrition education, nutrition counseling, coordination of nutrition care

Typically used to determine and to monitor and evaluate change in the following nutrition diagnoses: Inadequate energy intake, excessive energy intake, evident protein-calorie malnutrition, inadequate protein-energy intake, underweight, involuntary weight loss, overweight/obesity, involuntary weight gain, swallowing difficulty, breastfeeding difficulty, altered GI function, limited adherence to nutrition-related recommendations

Clinical judgment must be used to select indicators and determine the appropriate measurement techniques and reference standards for a given patient population and setting. Once identified, these indicators, measurement techniques, and reference standards should be identified in policies and procedures or other documents for use in patient/client records, quality or performance improvement, or in formal research projects.

Evaluation

Criteria for Evaluation

Comparison to Goal or Reference Standard:

1) Goal (tailored to individual's needs)
   OR
2) Reference Standard (estimated or measured energy requirement)

4th Edition

Energy Intake (FH-1.1.1)

Patient/Client Example

Indicator(s) Selected
Total energy intake

Criteria for Evaluation
Comparison to Goal or Reference Standard:
1) Goal: Food diary indicates patient/client consumes approximately 2600 calories/kcal (10,885 kJ) per day. Patient/client's target calorie intake level is 1800 calories/ kcal (7540 kJ) per day.
OR
2) Reference Standard: Patient/client's I & O indicates patient/client's intake at approximately 2000 calories/kcal (8375kJ) per day, 80% of goal based on an estimated energy requirement of 2500 calories/kcal (10465 kJ) per day.

Sample Nutrition Assessment and Monitoring and Evaluation Documentation

Initial encounter with patient/client	Based on patient/client food diary, patient/client consuming approximately 2600 calories/kcal (10,885 kJ) per day, 144% of recommended level of 1800 calories/ kcal (7540 kJ) per day. Will evaluate calorie intake at next encounter in two weeks.
Reassessment after nutrition intervention	Significant progress toward meeting goal. Based on patient/client food diary, patient/client consuming approximately 2100 calories/kcal (8790 kJ) per day, 117% of recommended level of 1800 calories/ kcal (7540 kJ) per day. Will evaluate calorie intake at next encounter in two weeks.

Updated; 2013 Edition

Fluid/Beverage Intake (FH-1.2.1)

Definition

Amount and type of fluid/beverage intake consumed orally

> *Note: Whenever possible, nutrient intake data should be considered in combination with clinical, biochemical, anthropometric information, medical diagnosis, clinical status, and/ or other factors as well as diet to provide a valid assessment of nutritional status based on a totality of the evidence.* (Institute of Medicine. Dietary Reference Intakes: Applications *in Dietary Assessment. Washington, DC: National Academies Press; 2000.)*

Nutrition Assessment and Monitoring and Evaluation

Indicators

Oral fluid (specify, e.g., oz, or mL or cups/day and type)

- Water
- Coffee and tea
- Juice
- Milk
- Soda (specify regular or artificially sweetened)

Food-derived fluids (e.g., 3 oz (90 mL) fluid in 4 oz (120 mL) apple sauce) (mL/day)

Liquid meal replacement or supplement (e.g., oz, or mL/day and name description)

> *Note:Biochemical measures of hydration status are found on the Electrolyte and Renal Profile and the Urine Profile reference sheets.*

Examples of the measurement methods or data sources for these indicators: Food intake records, 24-hour recall, food frequency questionnaire, intake and output data, observation

Typically used with the following domains of nutrition interventions: Food and/or nutrient delivery, nutrition education, nutrition counseling, coordination of nutrition care

Typically used to determine and to monitor and evaluate change in the following nutrition diagnoses: Excessive or inadequate oral food/beverage intake, food–medication interaction, underweight, overweight/obesity, involuntary weight loss, involuntary weight gain, disordered eating pattern, undesirable food choices, limited adherence to nutrition-related recommendations, inability or lack of desire to manage self-care, swallowing difficulty, breastfeeding difficulty, altered GI function

Clinical judgment must be used to select indicators and determine the appropriate measurement techniques and reference standards for a given patient population and setting. Once identified, these indicators, measurement techniques, and reference standards should be identified in policies and procedures or other documents for use in patient/client records, quality or performance improvement, or in formal research projects.

Fluid/Beverage Intake (FH-1.2.1)

Evaluation

Criteria for Evaluation

Comparison to Goal or Reference Standard:
1) Goal (tailored to patient/client's needs)
   OR
2) Reference Standard

Patient/Client Example(s)

Example(s) of one or two of the Nutrition Care Indicators (includes sample initial and reassessment documentation for one of the indicators)

Indicator(s) Selected

Oral fluid amounts

Criteria for Evaluation

Comparison to Goal or Reference Standard:
1) Goal: Patient/client currently drinks 33 oz (1000 mL) of fluid per day and has a personal goal of consuming
   64 oz (1920 mL) of fluid per day.
   OR
2) Reference Standard: No validated standard exists.

Sample Nutrition Assessment and Monitoring and Evaluation Documentation

Initial nutrition assessment with patient/client	Based on patient/client food diary, patient/client consuming approximately 1000 mL fluid per day. Goal is to consume approximately 3000 mL/day. Will monitor fluid intake at next encounter.
Reassessment after nutrition intervention	Significant progress toward recommended fluid intake. Based on fluid intake records, patient/client increased consumption of fluids from 1000 mL to 2600 mL per day.

Updated: 2011 Edition

Food Intake (FH-1.2.2)

Definition

Amount, type, and pattern of food consumed and quality of diet

> *Note: Whenever possible, nutrient intake data should be considered in combination with clinical, biochemical, anthropometric information, medical diagnosis, clinical status, and/ or other factors as well as diet to provide a valid assessment of nutritional status based on a totality of the evidence. (*Institute of Medicine. Dietary Reference Intakes: Applications *in Dietary Assessment. Washington, DC: National Academies Press; 2000.)*

Nutrition Assessment and Monitoring and Evaluation
Indicators

Amount of food
- Grains (servings, cups/dL/mL, ounces/g)
- Fruits (servings/piece, cups/dL, ounces/g)
- Vegetables (servings/piece, cups/dL, ounces/g)
- Fruit and vegetable (servings/piece, cups/dL, ounces/g)
- Milk/milk products (servings, cups/dL/mL, ounce/g)
- Meat, poultry, fish, eggs, beans, nut products (servings/piece, cups/dL, ounces/g, teaspoon/tablespoon/mL)
- Fat and oils (servings, teaspoons/mL/g)
- Concentrated sweets (servings, ounces/g)
- Percent total meal eaten (percent)

Types of food/meals
- Fortified/enriched foods (specify, e.g., amount or servings calcium-fortified orange juice)
- Special dietary products or foods (specify, e.g., servings/day or week, and type, e.g., non-nutritive sweeteners, lactose-free, gluten-free)
- Ready to eat food selections (e.g., type and number/day or week)
- Convenience frozen meals (e.g., type and number/day or week)
- Self-prepared foods/snacks (specify type e.g., low or high in sodium, fat, fiber)

Meal/snack* pattern
- Number of meals (number/day)
- Number of snack(s) (number/day)

Diet (food and beverages) Quality Index
- Healthy Eating Index (HEI)
- Children's Diet Quality Index (C-DQI)
- Revised Children's Diet Quality Index (RC-DQI)
- Other (specify)

Food variety (present/absent)

> *Note: Liquid meal replacements/supplements are found on the Fluid Intake reference sheet.*
>   * *Snack is defined as food served between regular meals.*

Food Intake (FH-1.2.2)

Examples of the measurement methods or data sources for these indicators:
Food intake records, 24-hour recall, food frequency questionnaire, menu analysis, dietary and physical activity assessment tool (e.g., MyPlate SuperTracker), diet quality index (e.g., Healthy Eating Index, C-DQI, RC-DQI) or other reference intake standard tool

Typically used with the following domains of nutrition interventions: Food and/or nutrient delivery, nutrition education, nutrition counseling, coordination of nutrition care

Typically used to determine and to monitor and evaluate change in the following nutrition diagnoses: Excessive or inadequate oral food/beverage intake, food–medication interaction, underweight, overweight/obesity, disordered eating pattern, involuntary weight gain, involuntary weight loss, undesirable food choices, limited adherence to nutrition-related recommendations, inability or lack of desire to manage self-care, limited access to food, intake of unsafe food, inadequate or excessive energy, macronutrient or micronutrient intake

Clinical judgment must be used to select indicators and determine the appropriate measurement techniques and reference standards for a given patient population and setting. Once identified, these indicators, measurement techniques, and reference standards should be identified in policies and procedures or other documents for use in patient/client records, quality or performance improvement, or in formal research projects.

Evaluation

Criteria for Evaluation
Comparison to Goal or Reference Standard:
1) Goal (tailored to patient/client needs)
   OR
2) Reference Standard

Patient/Client Example(s)
Example(s) of one or two of the Nutrition Care Indicators (includes sample initial and reassessment documentation for one of the indicators)

Indicator(s) Selected
Amount of food

Criteria for Evaluation
Comparison to Goal or Reference Standard:
1) Goal: Patient/client currently eats approximately 1 to 2 servings of fruits and vegetables per day. Goal is to increase fruit and vegetable intake to 5 servings per day.
   OR
2) Reference Standard: Patient/client's current intake of 1 to 2 servings of fruits and vegetables per day is below the DASH Eating Plan recommendation of 9 servings of fruits and vegetables per day.

Food Intake (FH-1.2.2)

Sample Nutrition Assessment and Monitoring and Evaluation Documentation

Initial nutrition assessment with patient/client	Based on patient/client recall, patient/client consuming approximately 1 to 2 servings of fruits and vegetables per day. Will monitor fruit and vegetable intake at next encounter.
Reassessment after nutrition intervention	Some progress toward goal of 9 servings of fruits and vegetables per day. Based on food records, patient/client increased consumption of fruits and vegetables from approximately 1 to 4 servings per day.

Updated: 2013 Edition

Breastmilk*/Infant Formula Intake (FH-1.2.3)

Definition
Amount of breastmilk, and/or the amount, type, and concentration on infant formula consumed orally

Nutrition Assessment and Monitoring and Evaluation
Indicators
Breastmilk intake (adequacy or oz or mL/day, mL/kg, percent recommended intake)
- Number of feedings (feedings/24-hour period)
- Duration of feedings (number of minutes)
- Modifier/supplement (specify, e.g., thickener, lipid, formula, protein)

Infant formula intake (oz or mL/day)
- Type (specify, e.g., brand, cow's milk-based, soy-based, preterm formula, or other specialty with or
  without DHA and ARA)
- Concentration (specify, e.g., calorie, kcal or kJ/oz or calorie, kcal or kJ /mL)
- Number of feedings (number/day)
- Volume of formula per feeding (oz or mL; amount prepared – amount left in bottle)
- Number and volume or weight of cans of formula used per week (powder, liquid concentrate,
  or ready to feed)
- Modifier/supplement (specify, e.g., thickener, lipid, formula, protein)

> *Note: Initiation, duration, exclusivity of breastfeeding and breastfeeding problems can be found on the Breastfeeding reference sheet.*
>
> *Weight change is found on the Body Composition/Growth/Weight History reference sheet.*
>
> *Number of wet diapers per day is found on the Urine Profile reference sheet.*
>
> *Number/consistency of bowel movements is found on the Nutrition-Focused Physical Exam reference sheet.*
>
> *If provided via tube use the Enteral and Parenteral Nutrition Intake reference sheet.*

Examples of the measurement methods or data sources for these indicators:
Intake records, 24-hour recall, usual intake recall, observation of feeding (bottle or breast).

Typically used with the following domains of nutrition interventions: Food and/or nutrient delivery, nutrition education, nutrition counseling, coordination of nutrition care

*If a synonym for the term "breastmilk" is helpful or needed, an approved alternate is "human milk."

Breastmilk/Infant Formula Intake (FH-1.2.3)

Typically used to determine and to monitor and evaluate change in the following nutrition diagnoses: Underweight, overweight, involuntary weight gain, involuntary weight loss, limited adherence to nutrition-related recommendations, inadequate or excessive energy intake, inadequate or excessive food/beverage or fluid intake

Clinical judgment must be used to select indicators and determine the appropriate measurement techniques and reference standards for a given patient population and setting. Once identified, these indicators, measurement techniques, and reference standards should be identified in policies and procedures or other documents for use in patient/client records, quality or performance improvement, or in formal research projects.

Evaluation

Criteria for Evaluation
Comparison to Goal or Reference Standard:
>   1) Goal (tailored to patient/client needs)
>   OR
>   2) Reference Standard

Patient/Client Example(s)
Example(s) of one or two of the Nutrition Care Indicators (includes sample initial and reassessment documentation for one of the indicators)

Indicator(s) Selected
Infant formula intake

Criteria for Evaluation
Comparison to Goal or Reference Standard:
>   1) Goal: Patient/client currently consumes approximately 100 mL/kg body weight infant formula per day. Goal is to increase intake to 150 mL/kg per day.
>   OR
>   2) Reference Standard: Patient/client's current intake of 100 mL/kg/day day is below the recommended intake of 150 mL/kg/day to support adequate growth.

Sample Nutrition Assessment and Monitoring and Evaluation Documentation

Initial nutrition assessment with patient/client	Based on mother's recall, patient/client consuming approximately 100 mL/kg/day of infant formula per day, 33% below the recommended level of 150 mL per day. Will monitor formula intake at next encounter.
Reassessment after nutrition intervention	Significant progress toward goal of consuming 150 mL/kg per day. Based on mother's records, patient/client increased consumption of infant formula to approximately 140 mL/kg per day over the past 7 days.

Enteral Nutrition Intake (FH-1.3.1)

Definition
Amount or type of enteral nutrition provided via a tube.

> *Note: Whenever possible, nutrient intake data should be considered in combination with clinical, biochemical, anthropometric information, medical diagnosis, clinical status, and/ or other factors as well as diet to provide a valid assessment of nutritional status based on a totality of the evidence.* (Institute of Medicine. Dietary Reference Intakes: Applications in Dietary Assessment. Washington, DC: National Academies Press; 2000.)

Nutrition Assessment and Monitoring and Evaluation
Indicators
Formula/solution (specify)
- Composition (formula name or description, special additives including supplemental fat, carbohydrate, protein fiber or other (specify)
- Concentration (e.g., calories/kcal/kJ in each mL)
- Rate (e.g., mL/hour)
- Volume, (e.g., mL/day, mL/hr, mL/feeding)
- Schedule, (e.g., number of hours per 24 hours, continuous, intermittent, bolus)

Feeding tube flush, e.g., type, volume, mL/flush, frequency

> *Note: Enteral nutrition tolerance can be accomplished with the Physical Exam reference sheet and/or the pertinent biochemical/sign or symptom reference sheet.*

Examples of the measurement methods or data sources for these indicators:
Patient/client report/recall, patient/client record, home evaluation, intake and output record

Typically used with the following domains of nutrition interventions: Food and/or nutrient delivery, nutrition education, coordination of nutrition care

Typically used to determine and to monitor and evaluate change in the following nutrition diagnoses: Inadequate or excessive intake of enteral nutrition, inadequate fluid intake, food–medication interaction, involuntary weight loss or gain

Clinical judgment must be used to select indicators and determine the appropriate measurement techniques and reference standards for a given patient population and setting. Once identified, these indicators, measurement techniques, and reference standards should be identified in policies and procedures or other documents for use in patient/client records, quality or performance improvement, or in formal research projects.

Evaluation

Criteria for Evaluation
Comparison to Goal or Reference Standard:
1) Goal (tailored to patient/client needs)
   OR
2) Reference Standard

Enteral Nutrition Intake (FH-1.3.1)

Patient/Client Example

Example(s) of one or two of the Nutrition Care Indicators (includes sample initial and reassessment documentation for one of the indicators)

Indicator(s) Selected

Rate/schedule (mL/hour × number of hours)

Criteria for Evaluation

Comparison to Goal or Reference Standard:

1) Goal: Patient/client's enteral nutrition is at a rate of 50 mL per hour × 24 hours of 1 calorie or kcal per mL formula compared to the nutrition prescription of 80 mL/hour × 24 hours to meet estimated nutrition requirements.

   OR

2) Reference Standard: There is no reference standard for this outcome because the provision of EN/PN is individualized.

Sample Nutrition Assessment and Monitoring and Evaluation Documentation

Initial nutrition assessment with patient/client	Enteral nutrition rate of 25 mL per hour × 24 hours of 1 calorie or kcal per mL formula compared to the nutrition prescription of 80 mL/hour to meet estimated nutrition requirements. Monitor enteral nutrition initiation and rate advancement.
Reassessment after nutrition intervention	Enteral nutrition at 70 mL per hour × 24 hours. Significant progress toward nutrition prescription of 1 calorie or kcal per mL formula at 80 mL per hour × 24 hours.

Updated: 2013 Editon

Parenteral Nutrition/IV Fluid Intake (FH-1.3.2)

Definition

Amount or type of parenteral nutrition and/or fluids provided intravenously.

> *Note: Whenever possible, nutrient intake data should be considered in combination with clinical, biochemical, anthropometric information, medical diagnosis, clinical status, and/or other factors as well as diet to provide a valid assessment of nutritional status based on a totality of the evidence. (Institute of Medicine.* Dietary Reference Intakes: Applications in Dietary Assessment. *Washington, DC: National Academies Press; 2000.)*

Nutrition Assessment and Monitoring and Evaluation

Indicators

Formula/solution (specify)
- Composition (formula or description)
- Concentration (e.g., percent, grams of solute per mL)
- Rate (e.g., mL/hour)
- Schedule (e.g., hours, timing, taper schedule)

Intravenous fluids, e.g., type; amount mL/day, mL/hr, mL with medications

> *Note: Parenteral nutrition tolerance can be accomplished with the Physical Exam Reference sheet and/or the pertinent biochemical/sign or symptom reference sheet.*

Examples of the measurement methods or data sources for these indicators:
Patient/client report/recall, patient/client record, home evaluation, intake and output record

Typically used with the following domains of nutrition interventions: Food and/or nutrient delivery, nutrition education, coordination of nutrition care

Typically used to determine and to monitor and evaluate change in the following nutrition diagnoses: Inadequate or excessive intake of parenteral nutrition, inadequate fluid intake, food–medication interaction, involuntary weight loss or gain

Clinical judgment must be used to select indicators and determine the appropriate measurement techniques and reference standards for a given patient population and setting. Once identified, these indicators, measurement techniques, and reference standards should be identified in policies and procedures or other documents for use in patient/client records, quality or performance improvement, or in formal research projects.

Evaluation

Criteria for Evaluation

Comparison to Goal or Reference Standard:
1) Goal (tailored to patient/client needs)
   OR
2) Reference Standard

Parenteral Nutrition/IV Fluid Intake (FH-1.3.2)

Patient/Client Example
Example(s) of one or two of the Nutrition Care Indicators (includes sample initial and reassessment documentation for one of the indicators)

Indicator(s) Selected
Rate/schedule (mL/hour × number of hours)

Criteria for Evaluation
Comparison to Goal or Reference Standard:

1) Goal: Patient/client's parenteral nutrition is at a rate of 50 mL per hour × 24 hours of standard solution compared to the nutrition prescription of 80 mL/hour × 24 hours to meet estimated nutrition requirements.
   OR
2) Reference Standard: There is no reference standard for this outcome as the provision of EN/PN is individualized.

Sample Nutrition Assessment and Monitoring and Evaluation Documentation

Initial nutrition assessment with patient/client	Parenteral nutrition rate of 25 mL per hour × 24 hours of standard solution compared to the nutrition prescription of 80 mL/hour to meet estimated nutrition requirements. Monitor nutrition initiation and rate advancement.
Reassessment after nutrition intervention	Parenteral nutrition at 70 mL per hour × 24 hours. Significant progress toward nutrition prescription of 80 mL per hour × 24 hours.

Updated: 2013 Editon

Alcohol Intake (FH-1.4.1)

Definition
Amount and pattern of alcohol consumption

Nutrition Assessment and Monitoring and Evaluation
Indicators
Drink size/volume (oz or mL)

Frequency (drinks/day and/or number of drinking days per week)

Pattern of alcohol consumption (number/size of drinks on drinking days)

Note: 1 drink = 5 oz (150mL) wine, 12 oz (350mL) beer, 1.5 oz (45mL) distilled alcohol

Examples of the measurement methods or data sources for these indicators: Patient/client report/recall, self-monitoring log

Typically used with the following domains of nutrition interventions: Nutrition education, nutrition counseling

Typically used to determine and to monitor and evaluate change in the following nutrition diagnoses: Excessive intake of alcohol; excessive or inadequate intake of energy; altered nutrition-related laboratory values; impaired nutrient utilization; overweight/obesity

Clinical judgment must be used to select indicators and determine the appropriate measurement techniques and reference standards for a given patient population and setting. Once identified, these indicators, measurement techniques, and reference standards should be identified in policies and procedures or other documents for use in patient/client records, quality or performance improvement, or in formal research projects.

Evaluation

Criteria for Evaluation
Comparison to Goal or Reference Standard:
1) Goal (tailored to patient/client needs)
   OR
2) Reference Standard

Patient/Client Example
Example(s) of one or two of the Nutrition Care Indicators (includes sample initial and reassessment documentation for one of the indicators)

Indicator(s) Selected
Pattern of alcohol consumption (number/size of drinks on drinking days)

Alcohol Intake (FH-1.4.1)

Criteria for Evaluation

Comparison to Goal or Reference Standard:

1) Goal: Patient/client's intake of one, 5 oz (150 mL) glass of wine 2 to 3 times per week is significantly above and non-compliant with the goal to abstain from alcohol during pregnancy.

   OR

2) Reference Standard: Patient/client's intake of three to four, 5 oz (150 mL) glasses of wine on drinking days is significantly above (above or consistent with) the recommendation of one 5 oz (150 mL) glass of wine per day for adult females.

Sample Nutrition Assessment and Monitoring and Evaluation Documentation

Initial nutrition assessment with patient/client	Based on recall, patient/client consuming three to four 5 oz (150 mL) glasses of wine on drinking days, which is above the recommended amount for females. Will monitor change in alcohol intake at next encounter.
Reassessment after nutrition intervention	Progress toward reference standard of up to one 5 oz (150 mL) glass of wine per day. Based on 7-day record, patient/client consuming 3 oz (90 mL) of wine on drinking days.

Bioactive Substance Intake (FH-1.4.2)

Definition
Amount and type of bioactive substances consumed

> *Note: Bioactive substances are not part of the Dietary Reference Intakes, and therefore there are no established minimum requirements or Tolerable Upper Intake Levels. However, RDs can assess whether estimated intakes are adequate or excessive using the patient/client goal or nutrition prescription for comparison.*

> *Working definition of bioactive substances—physiologically active components of foods that may have an effect on health. There is no scientific consensus about a definition for bioactive substances/components.*

Nutrition Assessment and Monitoring and Evaluation
Indicators
    Plant stanol esters (grams/day)

    Plant sterol esters (grams/day)

    Soy protein (grams/day)

    Psyllium (grams/day)

    β-glucan (grams/day)

    Food additives (those thought to have an impact on a patient/client's health), specify

    Other, specify

Examples of the measurement methods or data sources for these indicators:
Patient/client report/recall, self-monitoring log

Typically used with the following domains of nutrition interventions: Nutrition education, nutrition counseling

Typically used to determine and to monitor and evaluate change in the following nutrition diagnoses: Inadequate or excessive intake of bioactive substances, food–medication interaction

Clinical judgment must be used to select indicators and determine the appropriate measurement techniques and reference standards for a given patient population and setting. Once identified, these indicators, measurement techniques, and reference standards should be identified in policies and procedures or other documents for use in patient/client records, quality or performance improvement, or in formal research projects.

Evaluation

Criteria for Evaluation
Comparison to Goal or Reference Standard:
    1) Goal (tailored to patient/client needs)
        OR
    2) Reference Standard

Bioactive Substance Intake (FH-1.4.2)

Patient/Client Example
Example(s) of one or two of the Nutrition Care Indicators (includes sample initial and reassessment documentation for one of the indicators)

Indicator(s) Selected
Plant sterol and/or stanol esters (grams/day)

Criteria for Evaluation
Comparison to Goal or Reference Standard:
1) Goal: The patient/client does not consume plant sterol or stanol esters compared to the goal intake of 2 to 3 grams per day.
   OR
2) Reference Standard: No validated standard exists.

Sample Nutrition Assessment and Monitoring and Evaluation Documentation

Initial assessment with patient/client	Based on recall, patient/client not consuming (0 grams) stanol and/or sterol esters per day, which is below the goal intake of 2 to 3 grams per day. Will monitor change in stanol/sterol ester intake at next encounter.
Reassessment after nutrition intervention	Good progress toward the goal of 2 to 3 grams per day of stanol and/or sterol ester. Based on 7-day diet record, patient/client consuming 2 to 3 grams stanol/sterol ester per day, 2 to 3 days per week.

Updated: 2013 Edition

Caffeine Intake (FH-1.4.3)

Definition

Amount of caffeine intake from all sources, e.g., food, beverages, supplements, medications, and via enteral and parenteral routes

Nutrition Assessment and Monitoring and Evaluation

Indicators

Total caffeine intake (mg/day, e.g. naturally occurring caffeine in leaves, seeds, fruits of plants and sources with added caffeine such as water/beverages, medications)

Examples of the measurement methods or data sources for these indicators:
Patient/client report/recall, self-monitoring log

Typically used with the following domains of nutrition interventions: Nutrition education, nutrition counseling

Typically used to determine and to monitor and evaluate change in the following nutrition diagnoses: Food and nutrition-related knowledge deficit

Clinical judgment must be used to select indicators and determine the appropriate measurement techniques and reference standards for a given patient population and setting. Once identified, these indicators, measurement techniques, and reference standards should be identified in policies and procedures or other documents for use in patient/client records, quality or performance improvement, or in formal research projects.

Evaluation

Criteria for Evaluation

Comparison to Goal or Reference Standard:
1) Goal (tailored to patient/client needs)
   OR
2) Reference Standard

Patient/Client Example

Example(s) of one or two of the Nutrition Care Indicators (includes sample initial and reassessment documentation for one of the indicators)

Indicator(s) Selected

Total caffeine intake (mg/day)

Criteria for Evaluation

Comparison to Goal or Reference Standard:
1) Goal: The patient/client's intake is 600 mg of caffeine per day, which is above the goal of < 300 mg caffeine/day.
   OR
2) Reference Standard: The patient/client's intake is approximately 600 mg of caffeine/day which is above (above, below, or consistent with) of the reference standard of 400 mg caffeine/day.

Caffeine Intake (FH-1.4.3)

Sample Nutrition Assessment and Monitoring and Evaluation Documentation

Initial assessment with patient/client	Based on recall, patient/client consuming approximately 600 mg caffeine/day, which is above the reference standard of 400 mg/day. Will monitor change in caffeine intake at next encounter.
Reassessment after nutrition intervention	No progress toward the reference standard of 400 mg caffeine/day. Based on 3-day diet record, patient/client still consuming 600 mg caffeine/day.

Fat and Cholesterol Intake (FH-1.5.1)

Definition

Fat and cholesterol consumption from all sources, e.g., food, beverages, supplements, and via enteral and parenteral routes

> *Note: Whenever possible, nutrient intake data should be considered in combination with clinical, biochemical, anthropometric information, medical diagnosis, clinical status, and/ or other factors as well as diet to provide a valid assessment of nutritional status based on a totality of the evidence.* (Institute of Medicine. Dietary Reference Intakes: Applications *in Dietary Assessment. Washington, DC: National Academies Press; 2000.)*

Nutrition Assessment and Monitoring and Evaluation

Indicators

Total fat (specify, e.g., grams/day, grams/kg/day, percentage of calories, kcal or kJ)

Saturated fat (specify, e.g., grams/day or percentage of calories, kcal or kJ/day)

Trans fatty acids (specify, e.g., grams/day or percentage of calories, kcal or kJ/day)

Polyunsaturated fat (specify, e.g., grams/day or percentage of calories, kcal or kJ/day)

Monounsaturated fat (specify, e.g., grams/day or percentage of calories, kcal or kJ/day)

Omega-3 fatty acids
- Marine-derived (specify, e.g., grams/day)
- Plant-derived
    - Alpha-linolenic acid (specify, e.g., grams/day or percentage of calories, kcal or kJ/day)

Dietary cholesterol (specify, e.g., mg/day)

Essential fatty acids (specify, e.g., grams or ratio)

> *Note:Plant sterol and stanol esters can be found on the Bioactive Substance Intake Reference sheet.*

Examples of the measurement methods or data sources for these indicators:
Food intake records, 24-hour recall, food frequency questionnaires, menu analysis, fat and cholesterol targeted questionnaires and monitoring devices

Typically used with the following domains of nutrition interventions: Food and/or nutrient delivery, nutrition education, nutrition counseling

Typically used to determine and to monitor and evaluate change in the following nutrition diagnoses: Inadequate and excessive fat intake, less-than-optimal intake of types of fats, overweight/obesity, altered nutrition-related lab values, altered food and nutrition-related knowledge deficit

Fat and Cholesterol Intake (FH-1.5.1)

Clinical judgment must be used to select indicators and determine the appropriate measurement techniques and reference standards for a given patient population and setting. Once identified, these indicators, measurement techniques, and reference standards should be identified in policies and procedures or other documents for use in patient/client records, quality or performance improvement, or in formal research projects.

Evaluation

Criteria for Evaluation

Comparison to Goal or Reference Standard:
1) Goal (tailored to patient/client's needs)
   OR
2) Reference Standard

Patient/Client Example(s)

Example(s) of one or two of the Nutrition Care Indicators (includes sample initial and reassessment documentation for one of the indicators)

Indicator(s) Selected

Total fat (percentage of calories, kcal or kJ from fat)

Criteria for Evaluation

Comparison to Goal or Reference Standard:
1) Goal: Patient/client currently consumes 40% of calories, kcal or kJ from fat. Goal is to decrease fat intake to 25 to 35% of calories, kcal or kJ.
   OR
2) Reference Standard: Patient/client's intake of 350 mg of cholesterol per day is 175% of the National Heart, Lung and Blood Institute, Adult Treatment Panel III guidelines of less than 200 mg of dietary cholesterol per day.

Sample Nutrition Assessment and Monitoring and Evaluation Documentation

Initial nutritional assessment with patient/client	Based on a three-day food diary, patient/client is consuming approximately 40% of calories, kcal or kJ from fat. Patient/client goal is to reduce total fat intake to 25 to 35% of calories, kcal or kJ. Will monitor fat and calorie intake at next appointment.
Reassessment after nutrition intervention	Significant progress toward the goal intake of 25 to 35% calories, kcal or kJ from fat. Based on a three-day food diary patient/client's total fat intake decreased from approximately 40% to 38% calories, kcal or kJ from fat/day. Will continue to monitor progress at next encounter in 6 weeks.

Protein Intake (FH-1.5.2)

Definition
Protein intake from all sources, e.g., food, beverages, supplements, and via enteral and parenteral routes

> *Note: Whenever possible, nutrient intake data should be considered in combination with clinical, biochemical, anthropometric information, medical diagnosis, clinical status, and/ or other factors as well as diet to provide a valid assessment of nutritional status based on a totality of the evidence.* (Institute of Medicine. Dietary Reference Intakes: Applications *in Dietary Assessment. Washington, DC: National Academies Press; 2000.)*

Nutrition Assessment and Monitoring and Evaluation
Indicators
Total protein (specify, e.g., grams/day, grams/kg/day, percentage of calories, kcal or kJ)

High biological value protein (specify, e.g., grams/day, percentage of calories, kcal or kJ)

Casein (specify, e.g., grams/day)

Whey (specify, e.g., grams/day)

Amino acids (specify, e.g., percentage of crystalline amino acids)

Essential amino acids (specify, e.g., mg/day)

> *Note: Soy protein can be found on the Bioactive Substance Intake Reference sheet.*

Examples of the measurement methods or data sources for these indicators:
Food intake records, 24-hour recall, food frequency questionnaires, protein intake collection tools, nutrition fact labels, other product information, nutrient composition tables

Typically used with the following domains of nutrition interventions: Food and/or nutrient delivery, nutrition education, nutrition counseling, coordination of nutrition care

Typically used to determine and to monitor and evaluate change in the following nutrition diagnoses: Inadequate and excessive protein intake, less than optimal intake of types of proteins or amino acids, malnutrition, inadequate protein-energy intake, altered GI function, limited adherence to nutrition-related recommendations

Clinical judgment must be used to select indicators and determine the appropriate measurement techniques and reference standards for a given patient population and setting. Once identified, these indicators, measurement techniques, and reference standards should be identified in policies and procedures or other documents for use in patient/client records, quality or performance improvement, or in formal research projects.

Protein Intake (FH-1.5.2)

Evaluation

Criteria for Evaluation

Comparison to Goal or Reference Standard:

1) Goal (tailored to patient/client's needs)
   OR
2) Reference Standard

Patient/Client Example(s)

Example(s) of one or two of the Nutrition Care Indicators (includes sample initial and reassessment documentation for one of the indicators)

Indicator(s) Selected

Total protein

Criteria for Evaluation

Comparison to Goal or Reference Standard:

1) Goal: Patient/client's current intake of 25 g protein per day is below the recommended level of 55 to 65 g per day.
   OR
2) Reference Standard: (Used when patient goal is based on the population standard) Patient/client's intake of 12 g protein/day is less then the DRI of 53 g/day (0.8 g/kg BW). Patient/client's goal is to increase protein intake to approximately 55 g/day.

Sample Nutrition Assessment and Monitoring and Evaluation Documentation

Initial nutrition assessment with patient/client	Enteral feeding currently providing 25 g protein/day, well below the recommended level of 55 to 65 g/day (1 to 1.2 g/kg BW). Will continue to monitor protein intake daily.
Reassessment after nutrition intervention	Some progress toward goal intake of 55 to 65 g protein/day. Current intake approximately 30 g protein/day, 25 g protein below desired level. Will continue to monitor protein intake daily.

Carbohydrate Intake (FH-1.5.3)

Definition

Carbohydrate consumption from all sources, e.g., food, beverages, supplements, and via enteral and parenteral routes

> *Note: Whenever possible, nutrient intake data should be considered in combination with clinical, biochemical, anthropometric information, medical diagnosis, clinical status, and/ or other factors as well as diet to provide a valid assessment of nutritional status based on a totality of the evidence.* (Institute of Medicine. Dietary Reference Intakes: Applications *in Dietary Assessment. Washington, DC: National Academies Press; 2000.)*

Nutrition Assessment and Monitoring and Evaluation

Indicators

Total carbohydrate (specify, e.g., grams/day, grams/meal, grams/kg/min, percent of calories, kcal or kJ)

Sugar (specify, e.g., grams/day, percentage of calories, kcal or kJ)

Starch (specify, e.g., grams/day, percentage of calories, kcal or kJ)

Glycemic index (specify)

Glycemic load (specify)

Source of carbohydrate intake (food, beverage, tube feeding, parenteral nutrition, medication)

Insulin-to-carbohydrate ratio (specify)

> *Note: Fiber intake is listed on the Fiber Intake Reference sheet.*
>
> *Psyllium and β-glucan can be found on the Bioactive Substance Intake reference sheet.*

Examples of the measurement methods or data sources for these indicators:

Food intake records, 24-hour or typical day's recall, food frequency questionnaires, menu analysis, carbohydrate counting tools, intake/output sheets (for tube feeding or parenteral nutrition)

Typically used with the following domains of nutrition interventions: Food and/or nutrient delivery, nutrition education, nutrition counseling, coordination of nutrition care

Typically used to determine and to monitor and evaluate change in the following nutrition diagnoses: Inadequate and excessive carbohydrate intake, less-than-optimal intake of types of carbohydrate, inconsistent carbohydrate intake, altered nutrition-related laboratory values, food medication interaction

Clinical judgment must be used to select indicators and determine the appropriate measurement techniques and reference standards for a given patient population and setting. Once identified, these indicators, measurement techniques, and reference standards should be identified in policies and procedures or other documents for use in patient/client records, quality or performance improvement, or in formal research projects.

Carbohydrate Intake (FH-1.5.3)

Evaluation

Criteria for Evaluation

Comparison to Goal or Reference Standard:

    1) Goal (tailored to patient/client's needs)
       OR
    2) Reference Standard

Patient/Client Example(s)

Example(s) of one or two of the Nutrition Care Indicators (includes sample initial and reassessment documentation for one of the indicators)

Indicator(s) Selected

Total carbohydrate (distribution by meal)

Criteria for Evaluation

Comparison to Goal or Reference Standard:

    1) Goal: Patient/client's current carbohydrate intake in the morning ranges from 0 to 95 grams. The goal is that the patient/client will consume approximately 30 g carbohydrate at breakfast 6 days per week.
       OR
    2) Reference Standard: No validated standard exists.

Sample Nutrition Assessment and Monitoring and Evaluation Documentation

Initial nutrition assessment with patient/client	Based on carbohydrate counting tools, patient/client consumed 30 g carbohydrate at breakfast 2 days/week. Goal is to consume 30 g carbohydrate for breakfast 6 days per week.
Reassessment after nutrition intervention	Some progress made toward goal. Based on carbohydrate counting tools, patient/client consumed 30 g carbohydrate at breakfast 2 days/week. Will monitor breakfast carbohydrate intake at next encounter.

Updated: 2011 Edition

Fiber Intake (FH-1.5.4)

Definition

Amount and/or type of plant source matter consumed that is not completely digested, but may be at least partially fermented in the distal bowel, and is derived from all sources e.g., food, beverages, supplements, and via enteral routes

> *Note: Whenever possible, nutrient intake data should be considered in combination with clinical, biochemical, anthropometric information, medical diagnosis, clinical status, and/ or other factors as well as diet to provide a valid assessment of nutritional status based on a totality of the evidence. (*Institute of Medicine. Dietary Reference Intakes: Applications *in Dietary Assessment. Washington, DC: National Academies Press; 2000.)*

Nutrition Assessment and Monitoring and Evaluation

Indicators

Total fiber (g/day)

Soluble fiber (g/day)

Insoluble fiber (g/day)

- Fructooligosaccharides (g/day)

> *Note:Psyllium and β-glucan can be found on the Bioactive Substance Intake reference sheet*

Examples of the measurement methods or data sources for these indicators:

Food intake records, 24-hour recall, food frequency questionnaires, menu analysis, fiber counting tools, nutrition fact labels, other product information, nutrient composition tables

Typically used with the following domains of nutrition interventions: Food and/or nutrient delivery, nutrition education, nutrition counseling, coordination of nutrition care

Typically used to determine and to monitor and evaluate change in the following nutrition diagnoses: Inadequate and excessive fiber intake, altered GI function, disordered eating pattern, inadequate bioactive substance intake

Clinical judgment must be used to select indicators and determine the appropriate measurement techniques and reference standards for a given patient population and setting. Once identified, these indicators, measurement techniques, and reference standards should be identified in policies and procedures or other documents for use in patient/client records, quality or performance improvement, or in formal research projects.

Evaluation

Criteria for Evaluation

Comparison to Goal or Reference Standard:

1) Goal (tailored to patient/client's needs)
   OR
2) Reference Standard

Fiber Intake (FH-1.5.4)

Patient/Client Example(s)

Example(s) of one or two of the Nutrition Care Indicators (includes sample initial and reassessment documentation for one of the indicators)

Indicator(s) Selected

Total dietary fiber intake including those from foods and dietary fiber supplements.

Criteria for Evaluation

Comparison to Goal or Reference Standard:

1) Goal: Patient/client with current fiber intake of 15 g per day. Goal is to increase fiber intake to approximately 25 g per day.
   OR
2) Reference Standard: Patient/client's current intake of 15 g of dietary fiber per day is below the DRI of 25 g/day for a 40-year-old woman.

Sample Nutrition Assessment and Monitoring and Evaluation Documentation

Initial nutrition assessment with patient/client	Based on patient/client's food diary, patient/client is consuming approximately 15 g of fiber/day. Will monitor fiber intake at next encounter in three weeks.
Reassessment after nutrition intervention	Goal achieved. Patient/client's intake of 27 g fiber exceeded goal intake of 25 g/day. Will continue to monitor to ensure success is sustained.

Vitamin Intake (FH-1.6.1)

Definition
Vitamin intake from all sources, e.g., food, beverages, supplements, and via enteral and parenteral routes

> *Note: Whenever possible, nutrient intake data should be considered in combination with clinical, biochemical, anthropometric information, medical diagnosis, clinical status, and/ or other factors as well as diet to provide a valid assessment of nutritional status based on a totality of the evidence.* (Institute of Medicine. Dietary Reference Intakes: Applications in Dietary Assessment. Washington, DC: National Academies Press; 2000.)

Nutrition Assessment and Monitoring and Evaluation
Indicators
Vitamin A (specify form, µg or RE, frequency)

Vitamin C (mg, frequency)

Vitamin D (specify form, µg or IU, frequency)

Vitamin E (specify form, mg or IU, frequency)

Vitamin K (µg, frequency)

Thiamin (mg, frequency)

Riboflavin (mg, frequency)

Niacin (specify form, mg, frequency)

Vitamin B6 (specify form, mg, frequency)

Folate (specify form, µg, frequency)

Vitamin B12 (µg, frequency)

Pantothenic acid (mg, frequency)

Biotin (µg, frequency)

Multivitamin (yes/no, specify dose, frequency)

> *Note: Laboratory measures associated with body vitamin status can be found on the Vitamin Profile reference sheet.*

Examples of the measurement methods or data sources for these indicators:
Patient/client report or recall, food frequency, home evaluation, supplement use questionnaire

Typically used with the following domains of nutrition interventions: Food and/or nutrient delivery, nutrition education, nutrition counseling, coordination of nutrition care

Typically used to determine and to monitor and evaluate change in the following nutrition diagnoses: Excessive or inadequate intake of vitamins, parenteral, or enteral nutrition

Clinical judgment must be used to select indicators and determine the appropriate measurement techniques and reference standards for a given patient population and setting. Once identified, these indicators, measurement techniques, and reference standards should be identified in policies and procedures or other documents for use in patient/client records, quality or performance improvement, or in formal research projects.

Vitamin Intake (FH-1.6.1)

ASSESSMENT/MON & EVAL

Evaluation

Criteria for Evaluation

Comparison to Goal or Reference Standard:

1) Nutrition Prescription or Goal (tailored to patient/client needs)
   OR
2) Reference Standard

Patient/Client Example

Example(s) of one or two of the Nutrition Care Indicators (includes sample initial and reassessment documentation for one of the indicators)

Indicator(s) Selected

Vitamin D (µg or IU, frequency)

Criteria for Evaluation

Comparison to Goal or Reference Standard:

1) Nutrition Prescription or Goal: Use if patient/client's nutrition prescription/ goal is different from the reference standard.
   OR
2) Reference Standard: The patient/client's intake of 4 µg (160 IU) per day of Vitamin D is below (above, below, consistent with) the Adequate Intake (AI in the reference intake standard (e.g.,DRIs)) for males, age 14 to 18.

Sample Nutrition Assessment and Monitoring and Evaluation Documentation

Initial nutrition assessment with patient/client	Based on recall, patient/client with cystic fibrosis consuming approximately 4 µg for Vitamin D, which is below the Adequate Intake (AI) of 5 µg (200 IU) per day for Vitamin D for a 15-year-old male. Patient/client has also discontinued fat-soluble vitamin supplement. Will monitor Vitamin D intake at next encounter, intake of fat-soluble vitamin supplement, and request 25-Hydroxy, Vitamin D level (Vitamin Profile reference sheet).
Reassessment after nutrition intervention	25-Hydroxy, Vitamin D level below expected range (from Vitamin Profile). Significant progress toward the Adequate Intake of 5 µg (200 IU) for Vitamin D. Based on 3-day diet record, patient/client has increased consumption of Vitamin D from food sources to 5-7 µg (200-280 IU) for Vitamin D which is consistent with the Adequate Intake for healthy individuals, and is taking fat-soluble vitamin supplement on average 5 days per week. Despite meeting Adequate Intake, since patient/ client has cystic fibrosis, will need to continue fat-soluble vitamin supplementation in addition to food sources. Repeat lab in 3 months.

Updated: 2013 Edition

Mineral/Element Intake (FH-1.6.2)

Definition

Mineral/element intake from all sources, e.g., food, beverages, supplements, and via enteral and parenteral routes

> *Note: Whenever possible, nutrient intake data should be considered in combination with clinical, biochemical, anthropometric information, medical diagnosis, clinical status, and/ or other factors as well as diet to provide a valid assessment of nutritional status based on a totality of the evidence.* (Institute of Medicine. Dietary Reference Intakes: Applications in Dietary Assessment. Washington, DC: National Academies Press; 2000.)

Nutrition Assessment and Monitoring and Evaluation

Indicators

Calcium (specify form, mg, frequency)

Copper (µg or mg, frequency)

Fluoride (mg, frequency)

Iodine (µg, frequency)

Iron (specify form, mg, frequency)

Magnesium (mg, frequency)

Phosphorus (mg, frequency)

Manganese (mg, frequency)

Boron (mg, frequency)

Selenium (specify form, µg, frequency)

Zinc (mg, frequency)

Potassium (specify form, g or mg, frequency)

Sodium (mg or g, frequency)

Chloride (mg, frequency)

Chromium (specify form, µg, frequency)

Sulfate (g or mmol, frequency)

Molybdenum (µg, frequency)

Cobalt (µg, frequency)

Multi-mineral (yes/no, specify dose, frequency)

Multi-trace element (yes/no, specify dose, frequency)

Examples of the measurement methods or data sources for these indicators: Patient/client report or recall, food frequency, home evaluation, home care or pharmacy report, supplement use questionnaire

Typically used with the following domains of nutrition interventions: Food and/or nutrient delivery, nutrition education, nutrition counseling, coordination of nutrition care

Mineral/Element Intake (FH-1.6.2)

Typically used to determine and to monitor and evaluate change in the following nutrition diagnoses: Excessive or inadequate intake of minerals, food–medication interaction, altered nutrition-related laboratory values, impaired nutrient utilization, undesirable food choices, limited adherence to nutrition-related recommendations

Clinical judgment must be used to select indicators and determine the appropriate measurement techniques and reference standards for a given patient population and setting. Once identified, these indicators, measurement techniques, and reference standards should be identified in policies and procedures or other documents for use in patient/client records, quality or performance improvement, or in formal research projects.

Evaluation

Criteria for Evaluation
Comparison to Goal or Reference Standard:
1) Nutrition Prescription or Goal (tailored to individual's needs)
   OR
2) Reference Standard

Patient/Client Example
Example(s) of one or two of the Nutrition Care Indicators (includes sample initial and reassessment documentation for one of the indicators)

Indicator(s) Selected
Sodium (mg or g, frequency)
Calcium (specify form, mg, frequency)

Criteria for Evaluation
Comparison to Goal or Reference Standard:
1) Nutrition Prescription or Goal: The patient/client's intake of sodium is approximately 6000 mg per day, which is above the nutrition prescription of 4000 mg per day.
   OR
2) Reference Standard: The patient/client's intake of calcium is 500 mg per day which is 50% of the Adequate Intake (AI in the reference intake standard (e.g., DRIs)) for adult females, 31 to 50 years of age.

Sample Nutrition Assessment and Monitoring and Evaluation Documentation

Initial nutrition assessment with patient/client	Based on recall, patient/client consuming approximately 500 mg/day, which is below the adequate intake for calcium per day for females 31 to 50 years of age. Will monitor calcium intake at next encounter.
Reassessment after nutrition intervention	Significant progress toward the adequate intake of 1000 mg of calcium per day. Based on 3-day diet record, patient/client has increased consumption from 500 mg/day to 750 mg/day of the adequate daily intake for calcium.

Diet Order (FH-2.1.1)

Definition
A general or modified diet prescribed and documented in a patient/client medical record by a credentialed provider as part of a medical treatment plan

Nutrition Assessment
Indicators
General, healthful diet

Modified diet, specify, e.g., type, amount of energy and/or nutrients/day, distribution, texture

Enteral nutrition order, specify, e.g., formula, rate/schedule, access

Parenteral nutrition order, specify, e.g., solution, access, rate

Examples of the measurement methods or data sources for these indicators: Medical record, referring health care provider or agency, resident/client history

Typically used with the following domains of nutrition interventions: Food and/or nutrient delivery, nutrition education, nutrition counseling, coordination of nutrition care, resident/client history

Typically used with the following nutrition diagnoses: Inadequate or excessive energy, macronutrient or micronutrient intake, inadequate or excessive oral intake, swallowing difficulty

Clinical judgment must be used to select indicators and determine the appropriate measurement techniques and reference standards for a given patient population and setting. Once identified, these indicators, measurement techniques, and reference standards should be identified in policies and procedures or other documents for use in patient/client records, quality or performance improvement, or in formal research projects.

Evaluation

Criteria for Evaluation
Comparison to Goal or Reference Standard:
1) Goal (tailored to patient/client needs)
   OR
2) Reference Standard

Patient/Client Example(s)
Example(s) of one or two of the Nutrition Care Indicators (includes sample initial assessment documentation for one of the indicators)

Indicator(s) Selected
Modified diet

Diet Order (FH-2.1.1)

Criteria for Evaluation

Comparison to Goal or Reference Standard:

1) Goal: Not generally used

   OR

2) Reference Standard: No validated standard exists

Sample nutrition assessment documentation

Initial nutrition assessment with patient/client	Patient/client prescribed a 2,400 calorie or kcal (10,050 kJ) diabetic diet.

Updated: 2013 Edition

ASSESSMENT/MON & EVAL

Diet Experience (FH-2.1.2)

Definition
Previous nutrition/diet orders, diet education/counseling, and diet characteristics that influence patient/client's dietary intake

Nutrition Assessment
Indicators
Previously prescribed diets
- Previous modified diet (specify, e.g., type, amount of energy and/or nutrients/day, distribution, texture)
- Enteral nutrition order (specify)
- Parenteral nutrition order (specify)

Previous diet/nutrition education/counseling (specify, e.g., type, year)

Self-selected diets followed (specify, e.g., commercial diets, diet books, culturally directed)

Dieting attempts
- Number of past diet attempts (number)
- Results (specify, e.g., successful/unsuccessful, pounds or kg lost)
- Successful strategies (specify, e.g., no snacking, self-monitoring)

Food allergies
- Previous modified diet (specify, e.g., type and/or foods/food group) followed as a result of diagnosed or reported food allergy

Food intolerance
- Previous modified diet (specify, e.g., type and/or foods/food group) followed as a result of diagnosed or reported food intolerance

Examples of the measurement methods or data sources for these indicators:
Patient/client report, medical record, patient/client history, food and nutrition delivery coordination of care

Typically used with the following domains of nutrition interventions: Nutrition education, nutrition counseling

Typically used with the following nutrition diagnoses: Disordered eating pattern, not ready for diet/lifestyle change, excessive oral intake, food- and nutrition-related knowledge deficit, unsupported beliefs/attitudes about food- or nutrition-related topics, undesirable food choices, swallowing difficulty, intake of unsafe food

Clinical judgment must be used to select indicators and determine the appropriate measurement techniques and reference standards for a given patient population and setting. Once identified, these indicators, measurement techniques, and reference standards should be identified in policies and procedures or other documents for use in patient/client records, quality or performance improvement, or in formal research projects.

Diet Experience (FH-2.1.2)

Evaluation

Criteria for Evaluation

Comparison to Goal or Reference Standard:
1) Goal (tailored to patient/client needs)
   OR
2) Reference Standard

Patient/Client Example(s)

Example(s) of one or two of the Nutrition Care Indicators (includes sample initial assessment documentation for one of the indicators)

Indicator(s) Selected

Previous diet/nutrition education/counseling

Criteria for Evaluation

Comparison to Goal or Reference Standard:
1) Goal: Not generally used
   OR
2) Reference Standard: No validated standard exists

Sample nutrition assessment documentation

Initial nutrition assessment with patient/client	Patient/client completed a 6-week diabetic education class two years ago.

Updated: 2013 Edition

Eating Environment (FH-2.1.3)

Definition
The aggregate of surrounding things, conditions, or influences that affect food intake

Nutrition Assessment and Monitoring and Evaluation
Indicators
Location (specify, e.g., home, school, day care, restaurant, nursing home, senior center)

Atmosphere
- Acceptable noise level (yes/no)
- Appropriate lighting (yes/no)
- Appropriate room temperature (yes/no)
- Appropriate table height (yes/no)
- Appropriate table service (e.g., plates, napkins)/meal service (type of service, e.g., table service, buffet)/set-up (make food accessible for consumption) (yes/no)
- Eats at designated eating location (does not wander) (yes/no)
- Eats without distractions (e.g., watching TV/reading) (yes/no)
- No unpleasant odors (yes/no)

Caregiver/companion
- Allowed to select foods (often, sometimes, never)
- Caregiver influences/controls what client eats (e.g., encourages, forces) (yes/no)
- Caregiver models expected eating behavior (yes/no)
- Caretaker presence (present/not present)
- Favorite food is offered or withheld to influence behavior (reward/punishment) (yes/no)
- Has companionship while eating (another or others present) (yes/no)
- Meal/snacks offered at consistent times ("grazing" discouraged) (yes/no)

Appropriate breastfeeding accommodations/facility (yes/no)

Eats alone (specify reason, frequency)

Examples of the measurement methods or data sources for these indicators:
Patient/client report, medical record, referring health care provider or agency, observation

Typically used with the following domains of nutrition interventions: Food and/or nutrient delivery, nutrition education, nutrition counseling, coordination of nutrition care

Typically used to determine and to monitor and evaluate change in the following nutrition diagnoses: Inadequate oral intake, self-feeding difficulty, poor nutrition quality of life, limited access to food

Eating Environment (FH-2.1.3)

Clinical judgment must be used to select indicators and determine the appropriate measurement techniques and reference standards for a given patient population and setting. Once identified, these indicators, measurement techniques, and reference standards should be identified in policies and procedures or other documents for use in patient/client records, quality or performance improvement, or in formal research projects.

Evaluation

Criteria for Evaluation

Comparison to Goal or Reference Standard:

1) Goal (tailored to patient/client needs)
   OR
2) Reference Standard

Patient/Client Example(s)

Example(s) of one or two of the Nutrition Care Indicators (includes sample initial and reassessment documentation for one of the indicators)

Indicator(s) Selected

Eats at designated eating location

Criteria for Evaluation

Comparison to Goal or Reference Standard:

1) Goal: Two-year-old child with inadequate intake of calories/kcal/kJ and/ or nutrients. Goal is to improve intake through modifications in feeding environment and meal pattern.
   OR
2) Reference Standard: No validated standard exists

Sample Nutrition Assessment and Monitoring and Evaluation Documentation

Initial nutrition assessment with patient/client	Caregiver completed 3-day food record indicating multiple (10) feeding opportunities throughout the day. Child consumes mostly juice, dry cereal, and chips. Prefers foods that can be consumed from bottle or finger foods. Child does not sit at the table to eat, but wanders the house and is allowed to request and receive snacks ad lib. Energy and nutrient intake is less than 75% of standard. Referral to behavioral specialist offered.
Reassessment after nutrition intervention	Caregiver completed follow-up 3-day food record indicating reduced number of feeding opportunities throughout the day (6 to 7). States child resisted at first, but now eats at table at regular meal/snack times. Caregiver is continuing to work with behavioral specialist for both mealtime and other behavior issues. Energy and nutrient intake have improved to 85 to 90% of standard.

Enteral and Parenteral Nutrition Administration (FH-2.1.4)

Definition
Delivery of enteral and/or parenteral nutrition.

Nutrition Assessment and Monitoring and Evaluation
Indicators
Enteral access, specify, e.g., nasoentric, oroenteric, percutaneous, or surgical access with gastric, duodenal or jejunal placement

Parenteral access, specify, e.g., peripheral, central, and/or type of catheter

Body position, enteral nutrition (EN), specify, e.g., degree angle

Examples of the measurement methods or data sources for these indicators: Patient/client report/recall, patient/client record, patient/client nutrition-focused physical exam, provider referral

Typically used with following domains of nutrition interventions: Food and/or nutrient delivery, nutrition education, coordination of nutrition care

Typically used to determine the following nutrition diagnoses: Inadequate or excessive enteral or parenteral nutrition infusion, inadequate fluid intake, predicted food–medication interaction

Clinical judgment must be used to select indicators and determine the appropriate measurement techniques and reference standards for a given patient population and setting. Once identified, these indicators, measurement techniques, and reference standards should be identified in policies and procedures or other documents for use in patient/client records, quality or performance improvement, or in formal research projects.

Evaluation

Criteria for Evaluation
Comparison to Goal or Reference Standard:
1) Goal (tailored to patient/client's needs)
   OR
2) Reference Standard

Patient/Client Example(s)
Example(s) of one or two of the Nutrition Care Indicators (includes sample initial and reassessment documentation for one of the indicators)

Indicator(s) Selected
Enteral access (nasocentric)

Enteral and Parenteral Nutrition Administration (FH-2.1.4)

Criteria for Evaluation

Comparison to Goal or Reference Standard:

1) Goal: Patient/client's enteral nutrition is delieverd via nasoenteric feeding tube which will remain patent so patient/client can receive feeding to meet estimated nutrition requirements.

   OR

2) Reference Standard: There is no reference standard for this outcome.

Sample Nutrition Assessment and Monitoring and Evaluation Documentation

Initial nutrition assessment with patient/client	Patient/client's enteral nutrition is delieverd via nasoenteric feeding tube which will remain patent so patient/ client can receive feeding to meet estimated nutrition requirements. Monitor enteral nutrition feeding access for patency.
Reassessment after nutrition intervention	Enteral nutrition via nasoenteric feeding tube is blocked requiring replacement of feeding tube.

Updated: 2013 Edition

ASSESSMENT/MON & EVAL

Medications (FH-3.1)

Definition

Prescription and over-the-counter (OTC) medications that may impact nutritional status

Nutrition Assessment and Monitoring and Evaluation

Indicators

Prescription medication use
- Current prescriptions with nutrient/food–medication interactions, specify
- Insulin or insulin secretagogues, specify
- Medication, alter blood pressure, specify
- Medication, alter breastmilk production, specify
- Medication, lipid lowering, specify
- Medications, alter glucose levels, specify
- Other, specify

Over-the-counter (OTC) medications use
- Current OTC products with nutrient/food-medication implications, specify
- Medication, alter blood pressure, specify
- Medication, alter breastmilk production, specify
- Medication, lipid lowering, specify
- Medications, alter glucose levels, specify
- Other, specify

Misuse of medications (e.g., accidental overdose, illegal drugs, laxatives, diuretics, drug use during pregnancy), specify

Note: Vitamin and mineral supplements can be found on the vitamin and mineral intake reference sheets. Alcohol is found on the Alcohol Intake reference sheet

Examples of the measurement methods or data sources for these indicators:
Patient/client report, medical record, referring health care provider or agency

Typically used with following domains of nutrition interventions: Food and/or nutrient delivery, nutrition education, nutrition counseling, coordination of nutrition care

Typically used to determine the following nutrition diagnoses: Food–medication interaction, increased energy expenditure, malnutrition, inadequate or excessive energy, food/beverage, fluid, carbohydrate, protein, fat, vitamin and mineral intake, unintended weight gain or loss, overweight/obesity, underweight, disordered eating pattern

Clinical judgment must be used to select indicators and determine the appropriate measurement techniques and reference standards for a given patient population and setting. Once identified, these indicators, measurement techniques, and reference standards should be identified in policies and procedures or other documents for use in patient/client records, quality or performance improvement, or in formal research projects.

Medications (FH-3.1)

Evaluation

Criteria for Evaluation

Comparison to Goal or Reference Standard:

1) Goal (tailored to patient/client's needs)
   OR
2) Reference Standard

Patient/Client Example(s)

Example(s) of one or two of the Nutrition Care Indicators (includes sample initial and reassessment documentation for one of the indicators)

Indicator(s) Selected

Prescription medication with nutrient/food–medication interactions—Prednisone

Criteria for Evaluation

Comparison to Goal or Reference Standard:

1) Goal: Patient/client with prescription for 50 mg/d prednisone and concerned about concurrent weight gain caused by increased appetite and fluid retention. Goal is to minimize weight gain and maintain good nutritional status during prednisone therapy.
   OR
2) Reference Standard: Not applicable

Sample Nutrition Assessment and Monitoring and Evaluation Documentation

Initial nutrition assessment with patient/client	Patient/client's prescription medication is 50 mg/d prednisone for rheumatoid arthritis. Current weight 182 lb (83 kg). Long-term therapy may result in a need for protein, calcium, potassium, phosphorus, folate and vitamin A, C, and D supplementation. Patient/client currently taking a vitamin/mineral supplement and concerned about weight gain caused by increased appetite and fluid retention.
Reassessment after nutrition intervention	Patient/client's prescription medication prednisone dose reduced to 25 mg/d. Currently taking a one-a-day multivitamin/multimineral and snacking on raw vegetables between meals. Weight stable.

Updated: 2013 Edition

Complementary/Alternative Medicine (FH-3.2)

Definition
Complementary and alternative medicine products, including herbal preparations that may impact nutritional status

Nutrition Assessment and Monitoring and Evaluation
Indicators
Nutrition-related complementary/alternative medicine use (e.g., gingko, St. John's Wart, elderberry, garlic, ephedra)

> *Note: Vitamin and mineral supplements can be found on the vitamin and mineral intake reference sheets. Alcohol is found on the Alcohol Intake reference sheet*

Examples of the measurement methods or data sources for these indicators: Patient/client report, medical record, referring health care provider or agency

Typically used with following domains of nutrition interventions: Food and/or nutrient delivery, nutrition education, nutrition counseling, coordination of nutrition care

Typically used to determine the following nutrition diagnoses: Food–medication interaction, increased energy expenditure, malnutrition, unintended weight gain or loss, overweight/obesity, intake of unsafe foods, disordered eating pattern

Clinical judgment must be used to select indicators and determine the appropriate measurement techniques and reference standards for a given patient population and setting. Once identified, these indicators, measurement techniques, and reference standards should be identified in policies and procedures or other documents for use in patient/client records, quality or performance improvement, or in formal research projects.

Evaluation

Criteria for Evaluation
Comparison to Goal or Reference Standard:
1) Goal (tailored to patient/client's needs)
   OR
2) Reference Standard

Patient/Client Example(s)
Example(s) of one or two of the Nutrition Care Indicators (includes sample initial and reassessment documentation for one of the indicators)

Indicator(s) Selected
Complementary/alternative medicine use—ephedra

Complementary/Alternative Medicine (FH-3.2)

Criteria for Evaluation

Comparison to Goal or Reference Standard:

1) Goal: Patient/client taking ephedra with the hope that it will promote weight loss. Goal is to have patient/client eliminate ephedra for safety reasons and engage in nutrition counseling for weight management.
   OR
2) Reference Standard: Not applicable

Sample Nutrition Assessment and Monitoring and Evaluation Documentation

Initial nutrition assessment with patient/client	Patient/client complementary/alternative medicine use of ephedra is for weight loss. Patient/client reports being unaware of safety concerns.
Reassessment after nutrition intervention	Patient/client complementary/alternative medicine use of ephedra has stopped and success with weight loss as a result of nutrition counseling.

Created: 2013 Edition

Food and Nutrition Knowledge/Skill (FH-4.1)

Definition

Content areas and level of understanding about food, nutrition and health, or nutrition-related information and guidelines relevant to patient/client needs

Nutrition Assessment and Monitoring and Evaluation
Indicators

> Use the following terms to specify *level of knowledge/skill* by each area of concern:
> - *Inadequate*
> - *Basic* (survival, identify facts, little application)
> - *Moderate* (some application in typical situations)
> - *Comprehensive* (synthesize and evaluate for application in new situations)

Area(s) and level of knowledge/skill
- Breastfeeding (e.g., signs of infant satiety)
- Consequences of food behavior
- Disease/condition
- Goal-setting techniques
- Food label
- Food products
- Food/nutrient requirements
- Health knowledge gap (e.g., understanding of health or health guidance versus true health)
- Health care literacy
- Laboratory results compared to desirable
- Level of physical conditioning
- Nutrition recommendations
- Physiological functions
- Self-management parameters
- Control food portions
- Food preparation/cooking
- Manage behavior in response to stimuli (e.g., identify triggers/cues, develop a plan, modify environment or behavior)
- Plan meals/snacks
- Select healthful foods/meals
- Self-monitor
- Other (specify topic and level of knowledge)

Diagnosis specific or global nutrition-related knowledge score (specify instrument used, e.g., Type 2 Diabetes BASICS Pre/Post Knowledge Test and score)

Food and Nutrition Knowledge/Skill (FH-4.1)

Examples of the measurement methods or data sources for this indicator: Pre- and/or post-tests administered orally, on paper, or by computer, scenario discussions, patient/client restates key information, review of food records, practical demonstration/test, survey, nutrition quotient, nutrition questionnaire, nutrition assessment inventory

Typically used to determine and monitor and evaluate change in the following domains of nutrition interventions: Nutrition education, nutrition counseling

Typically used to determine and to monitor and evaluate change in the following nutrition diagnoses: Food- and nutrition-related knowledge deficit, limited adherence to nutrition-related recommendations, undesirable food choices, breastfeeding difficulty, overweight/obesity, intake domain

Clinical judgment must be used to select indicators and determine the appropriate measurement techniques and reference standards for a given patient population and setting. Once identified, these indicators, measurement techniques, and reference standards should be identified in policies and procedures or other documents for use in patient/client records, quality or performance improvement, or in formal research projects.

Evaluation

Criteria for Evaluation
Comparison to Goal or Reference Standard:
1) Goal (tailored to individual's needs)
   OR
2) Reference Standard

Patient/Client Example(s)
Example(s) of one or two of the Nutrition Care Indicators (includes sample initial and reassessment documentation for one of the indicators)

Indicator(s) Selected
Area and level of knowledge (carbohydrate counting)

Criteria for Evaluation
Comparison to Goal or Reference Standard:
1) Goal: Patient/client will be able to accurately read a food label and identify the total number of grams of carbohydrate per serving.
   OR
2) Reference Standard: No validated standard exists.

Food and Nutrition Knowledge/Skill (FH-4.1)

Sample Nutrition Assessment and Monitoring and Evaluation Documentation

Initial nutrition assessment with patient/client	Patient/client with newly diagnosed diabetes with inadequate knowledge regarding carbohydrate counting.
Reassessment after nutrition intervention	Patient/client with basic knowledge regarding carbohydrate counting. Able to apply knowledge to common scenarios, but not consistently able to apply knowledge to own diet. Will continue to monitor at next encounter in one week.

Updated: 2013 Edition

Beliefs and Attitudes (FH-4.2)

Definition

Conviction of the truth of some nutrition-related statement or phenomenon, and feelings or emotions toward that truth or phenomenon, along with a patient/client's readiness to change food, nutrition, or nutrition-related behaviors

Nutrition Assessment and Monitoring and Evaluation Indicators

Conflict with personal/family value system (specify)

Distorted body image (yes/no)

End-of-life decisions (specify)

Motivation
- Perceived susceptibility to nutrition-related health problems (e.g., patient/client believes he or she is diabetic or at high-risk for developing diabetes) (yes/no)
- Understanding of severity of risk to health/lifestyle (Perceived severity) (yes/no)
- Belief that benefits of diet change outweigh barriers (benefits are worth the sacrifice and effort) (yes/no)
- Verbalizes desire to change diet and nutrition-related behaviors (yes/no)

Preoccupation with food (yes/no)

Preoccupation with weight (yes/no)

Readiness to change nutrition-related behaviors
- Precontemplation (yes/no)
- Contemplation (yes/no)
- Preparation (yes/no)
- Action (yes/no)
- Maintenance (yes/no)

Self-efficacy
- Breastfeeding self-efficacy (specify, e.g., high, low)
- Eating self-efficacy (specify, e.g., high, low)
- Weight loss self-efficacy (specify, e.g., high, low)
- Other (specify)

Self-talk/cognitions (Documented cognitions related to food/nutrition activity) (positive/negative)

Unrealistic nutrition-related goals (specify, e.g., current weight loss goal of 20 lbs (9 kg)/month is unrealistic)

Unscientific beliefs/attitudes (specify, e.g., specific food with unsubstantiated curative power)

Food preferences (specify)

Emotions (specify, e.g., anger, guilt, sad, lonely, nervous)

ASSESSMENT/MON & EVAL

Beliefs and Attitudes (FH-4.2)

Examples of the measurement methods or data sources for these outcome indicators: Patient/client self-report, patient/client assessment questionnaire or interview, medical record, referring health care provider or agency

Typically used to monitor and evaluate change in the following domains of nutrition interventions: Nutrition education, nutrition counseling

Typically used to determine and to monitor and evaluate change in the following nutrition diagnoses: Unsupported beliefs/attitudes about food- or nutrition-related topics; not ready for diet/lifestyle change; inability to manage self-care; self-monitoring deficit, excessive or inadequate oral, energy, macronutrient, micronutrient or bioactive substance intake; imbalance of nutrients; less than optimal intake of types of fats; less than optimal intake of types of proteins or amino acids; underweight; overweight/obesity; disordered eating pattern; physical inactivity; excess physical activity; limited access to food and/or water

Clinical judgment must be used to select indicators and determine the appropriate measurement techniques and reference standards for a given patient population and setting. Once identified, these indicators, measurement techniques, and reference standards should be identified in policies and procedures or other documents for use in patient/client records, quality or performance improvement, or in formal research projects.

Evaluation

Criteria for Evaluation
Comparison to Goal or Reference Standard:
1) Goal (tailored to individual's needs)
   OR
2) Reference Standard

Patient/Client Example(s)
Example(s) of one or two of the Nutrition Care Indicators (includes sample initial and reassessment documentation for one of the indicators)

Indicator(s) Selected
Readiness to change nutrition-related behaviors

Criteria for Evaluation
Comparison to Goal or Reference Standard:
1) Goal: Patient/client is currently in the precontemplation stage of change. Patient/client goal is to move to the preparation stage of change within 3 months.
   OR
2) Reference Standard: No validated standard exists.

Beliefs and Attitudes (FH-4.2)

Sample Nutrition Assessment and Monitoring and Evaluation Documentation

Initial nutrition assessment with patient/client	Assessment results indicate patient/client is currently in the precontemplation stage of change related to need for DASH diet adherence. Will initiate motivational interviewing and reassess in two weeks.
Reassessment after nutrition intervention	Significant progress toward goal. Reassessment indicates that patient/client has moved from the precontemplation stage to the contemplation stage related to need for DASH diet adherence. Will reassess in two weeks.

Updated: 2011 Edition

Adherence (FH-5.1)

Definition

Level of compliance or adherence with nutrition-related recommendations or behavioral changes agreed upon by patient/client to achieve nutrition-related goals

Nutrition Assessment and Monitoring and Evaluation

Indicators

Self-reported adherence score (Rated on scale of 1 to 10; 1 = Not adherent, 10 = Completely adherent)

Nutrition visit attendance (ratio, number attended/total)

Ability to recall nutrition goals (full, partial, none)

Self-monitoring at agreed upon rate (Rated on scale of 1 to 10; 1 = Not adherent, 10 = Completely adherent)

Self-management based on details agreed upon (within the nutrition plan) (Rated on scale of 1 to 10; 1 = Not adherent, 10 = Completely adherent)

> *Note: Use in conjunction with appropriate Food and Nutrition Intake, Anthropometric Data, and Biochemical Data reference sheets.*
>
> *May be useful in relapse prevention treatment (analyze and control factors that caused the lapse).*

Examples of the measurement methods or data sources for these indicators: Nutrition visit attendance, self-monitoring records (e.g., to evaluate fat, sodium, calories/kcal/kJ, diet quality), patient/client self-report, adherence tools or questionnaires, provider assessment

Typically used with the following domains of nutrition interventions: Food and/or nutrient delivery, nutrition education, nutrition counseling

Typically used to determine and to monitor and evaluate change in the following nutrition diagnosis: Limited adherence to nutrition-related recommendations

Clinical judgment must be used to select indicators and determine the appropriate measurement techniques and reference standards for a given patient population and setting. Once identified, these indicators, measurement techniques, and reference standards should be identified in policies and procedures or other documents for use in patient/client records, quality or performance improvement, or in formal research projects.

Evaluation

Criteria for Evaluation

Comparison to Goal or Reference Standard:

1) Goal (tailored to individual's needs)
   OR
2) Reference Standard

Adherence (FH-5.1)

Patient/Client Example(s)

Example(s) of one or two of the Nutrition Care Indicators (includes sample initial and reassessment documentation for one of the indicators)

Indicator(s) Selected

Self-reported adherence score

Criteria for Evaluation

Comparison to Goal or Reference Standard:

1) Goal: Patient/client rates herself a 4 on a scale of 1 to 10 (1 = Not adherent, 10 = Completely adherent) on her level of adherence to nutrition-related goals. Patient/client desires to move to a rating of 8.
   OR
2) Reference Standard: No validated standard exists.

Sample nutrition assessment monitoring and evaluation documentation

Initial nutrition assessment with patient/client	Patient/client rates herself a 1 on a scale of 1 to 10 on her ability to adhere to her meal plan. Patient/client set a goal to adhere to her meal plan 5 days per week. Will evaluate adherence at the next encounter.
Reassessment after nutrition intervention	Some progress toward goal. Patient/client rated herself a 6 on a scale of 1 to 10 on her ability to meet her adherence goal of following her meal plan 5 days per week. Is doing well on weekdays, but states she must improve on weekends. Discussed ways to improve adherence to meal plan on the weekends. Will monitor at next encounter in two weeks.

ASSESSMENT/MON & EVAL

Avoidance Behavior (FH-5.2)

Definition

Keeping away from something or someone to postpone an outcome or perceived consequence

Nutrition Assessment and Monitoring and Evaluation

Indicators

Avoidance

- Specific foods (specify, e.g., grapefruit, seeds)
- Food groups (specify, e.g., milk/milk products)
- Fluids (specify)
- Textures (specify)
- Social situations (specify)
- Other (specify)

Restrictive eating (yes/no)

Cause of avoidance behavior (e.g., personal choice, prescribed dietary restriction, GI distress, suspected allergy, eating disorder, cancer treatment side effects, medications, mental illness, Parkinson's disease)

Examples of the measurement methods or data sources for these indicators: Self-monitoring records, patient/client interview

Typically used with the following domains of nutrition interventions: Nutrition counseling

Typically used to determine and to monitor and evaluate change in the following nutrition diagnoses: Disordered eating pattern, overweight/obesity, underweight, altered GI function

Clinical judgment must be used to select indicators and determine the appropriate measurement techniques and reference standards for a given patient population and setting. Once identified, these indicators, measurement techniques, and reference standards should be identified in policies and procedures or other documents for use in patient/client records, quality or performance improvement, or in formal research projects.

Evaluation

Criteria for Evaluation

Comparison to Goal or Reference Standard:

1) Goal (tailored to patient/client needs)
   OR
2) Reference Standard

Patient/Client Example(s)

Example(s) of one or two of the Nutrition Care Indicators (includes sample initial and reassessment documentation for one of the indicators)

Indicator(s) Selected

Avoidance of social situations

Avoidance Behavior (FH-5.2)

Criteria for Evaluation

Comparison to Goal or Reference Standard:

1) Goal: Patient/client avoiding social situations in an effort to avoid overeating. Goal is to learn strategies to control eating in social situations.

   OR

2) Reference Standard: No validated standard exists

Sample Nutrition Assessment and Monitoring and Evaluation Documentation

Initial nutrition assessment with patient/client	Patient/client avoids social situations because she is afraid she will overeat. Reviewed client's food diary and client brainstormed strategies which may help her control eating in social situations. Patient/client will preplan food intake on days she has social engagements, will have a piece of fruit before going to help curb her appetite and will maintain a food diary.
Reassessment after nutrition intervention	Patient/client made some progress toward goal. Attended 2 of 4 social engagements where food was served, and successfully controlled food intake both times. Patient/client will continue to use strategies. Will reevaluate avoidance behavior at next encounter.

Bingeing and Purging Behavior (FH-5.3)

Definition
Eating a larger amount of food than normal for the individual during a short period of time (within any two-hour period) accompanied by a lack of control over eating during the binge episode (i.e., the feeling that one cannot stop eating). This may be followed by compensatory behavior to make up for the excessive eating, referred to as purging.

Nutrition Assessment and Monitoring and Evaluation
Indicators
Binge eating behavior (present/absent)
- Number of binge episodes (e.g., number/day, number/week, number/month)

Purging behavior (present/absent)
- Self-induced vomiting (number/day, number/week, number/month)
- Fasting (yes/no)
- Other (specify)

> Note Misuse of laxatives, diuretics or other drugs is found on the Medication and Herbal Supplements reference sheet.
>
> Amount and type of physical activity is found on the Physical Activity reference sheet.

Examples of the measurement methods or data sources for these indicators: Patient/client interview, medical record, referring health care provider or agency, self-monitoring records

Typically used with following domains of nutrition interventions: Nutrition counseling

Typically used to determine and to monitor and evaluate change in the following nutrition diagnoses: Excessive oral food/beverage intake, disordered eating pattern, overweight/obesity

Clinical judgment must be used to select indicators and determine the appropriate measurement techniques and reference standards for a given patient population and setting. Once identified, these indicators, measurement techniques, and reference standards should be identified in policies and procedures or other documents for use in patient/client records, quality or performance improvement, or in formal research projects.

Evaluation

Criteria for Evaluation
Comparison to Goal or Reference Standard:
1) Goal (tailored to patient/client needs)
   OR
2) Reference Standard

Bingeing and Purging Behavior (FH-5.3)

Patient/Client Example(s)
Example(s) of one or two of the Nutrition Care Indicators (includes sample initial and reassessment documentation for one of the indicators)

Indicator(s) Selected
Number of binge episodes

Criteria for Evaluation
Comparison to Goal or Reference Standard:
1) Goal: Patient/client reports 3 binge eating episodes per week. Goal is to reduce binge eating to one episode per week.
   OR
2) Reference Standard: No validated standard exists.

Sample Nutrition Assessment and Monitoring and Evaluation Documentation

Initial encounter with patient/client	Patient/client reports 3 binge-eating episodes this week.
Reassessment after nutrition intervention	Some progress toward goal. Patient/client reported 2 binge eating episodes this week. Will continue to monitor at next encounter.

Mealtime Behavior (FH-5.4)

Definition
Manner of acting, participating, or behaving at mealtime which influences patient/client's food and beverage intake

Nutrition Assessment and Monitoring and Evaluation
Indicators
Meal duration (minutes)

Percent of meal time spent eating (percent)

Preference to drink rather than eat (yes/no)

Refusal to eat/chew (specify, e.g., meal, food type)

Spitting food out (specify, e.g., food type, frequency)

Rumination (yes/no)

Patient/client/caregiver fatigue during feeding process, resulting in inadequate intake (yes/no)

Willingness to try new foods (yes/no)

Limited number of accepted foods (specify)

Rigid sensory preferences (flavor, temperature, texture)

Examples of the measurement methods or data sources for these indicators: Observation, medical record, referring health care provider or agency, caregiver observation, patient/client interview

Typically used with following domains of nutrition interventions: Food and/or nutrient delivery, coordination of nutrition care

Typically used to determine and to monitor and evaluate change in the following nutrition diagnoses: Self-feeding difficulty, inadequate and excessive oral intake

Clinical judgment must be used to select indicators and determine the appropriate measurement techniques and reference standards for a given patient population and setting. Once identified, these indicators, measurement techniques, and reference standards should be identified in policies and procedures or other documents for use in patient/client records, quality or performance improvement, or in formal research projects.

Evaluation

Criteria for Evaluation
Comparison to Goal or Reference Standard:
1) Goal (tailored to patient/client needs)
   OR
2) Reference Standard

Patient/Client Example(s)
Example(s) of one or two of the Nutrition Care Indicators (includes sample initial and reassessment documentation for one of the indicators)

Mealtime Behavior (FH-5.4)

Indicator(s) Selected
Percent of meal spent eating (percentage)

Criteria for Evaluation
Comparison to Goal or Reference Standard:
1) Goal: Four-year-old patient/client with inadequate food/beverage intake. Lunch meal observation revealed less than 10% of mealtime was spent eating. Goal is to reduce environmental distractions and increase percent of meal spent eating to 55%.
   OR
2) Reference Standard: No validated standard exists

Sample Nutrition Assessment and Monitoring and Evaluation Documentation

Initial nutrition assessment with patient/client	Lunch meal observation revealed that patient/client is highly distracted and spends less than 10% of the mealtime eating.
Reassessment after nutrition intervention	Significant progress toward goal. Environmental distractions were minimized and caregiver eats meals with patient/client. Observation reveals that approximately 40% of mealtime is spent eating. Will monitor at next encounter.

ASSESSMENT/MON & EVAL

Social Network (FH-5.5)

Definition
Ability to build and utilize a network of family, friends, colleagues, health professionals, and community resources for encouragement, emotional support, and to enhance one's environment to support behavior change

Nutrition Assessment and Monitoring and Evaluation
Indicators
Ability to build and utilize social networks (e.g., may include perceived social support, social integration, and assertiveness)

Examples of the measurement methods used or data sources for these indicators: Self-monitoring records, client/patient self-report, goal-tracking tools

Typically used with the following domains of nutrition interventions: Nutrition counseling

Typically used to determine and to monitor and evaluate change in the following nutrition diagnoses: Intake domain, underweight, overweight/obesity, disordered eating pattern, undesirable food choices, inability to manage self-care, breastfeeding difficulty, not ready for diet/lifestyle change, limited adherence to nutrition-related recommendations

Clinical judgment must be used to select indicators and determine the appropriate measurement techniques and reference standards for a given patient population and setting. Once identified, these indicators, measurement techniques, and reference standards should be identified in policies and procedures or other documents for use in patient/client records, quality or performance improvement, or in formal research projects.

Evaluation

Criteria for Evaluation
Comparison to Goal or Reference Standard:
1) Goal (tailored to individual's needs)
   OR
2) Reference Standard

Patient/Client Example
Example(s) of one or two of the Nutrition Care Indicators (includes sample initial and reassessment documentation for one of the indicators)

Indicator(s) Selected
Ability to build and utilize social support (e.g., may include perceived social support, social integration, and assertiveness)

Social Network (FH-5.5)

Criteria for Evaluation

Comparison to Goal or Reference Standard:

1) Goal: Overweight patient/client's wife adds fat to all foods prepared at home. Goal is to reduce the amount of fat in meals prepared at home by asking wife to not dress the salad or add fat seasoning to vegetables before serving.

   OR

2) Reference Standard: No validated standard exists.

Sample Nutrition Assessment and Monitoring and Evaluation Documentation

Initial encounter with patient/client	Patient/client states that he rarely verbalizes his nutrition-related desires/needs in family or social situations and rates his ability to elicit social support a 3 on a scale of 1 to 10. Will evaluate at the next encounter.
Reassessment at a later date	Some progress toward goal. Patient/client rated himself a 5, on a scale of 1to10, on his ability to elicit social support. Has begun to verbalize his needs and plans to research restaurants that meet his needs that others will enjoy. Will monitor at next encounter in two weeks.

Food/Nutrition Program Participation (FH-6.1)

Definition
Patient/client eligibility for and participation in food assistance programs

Nutrition Assessment and Monitoring and Evaluation

Indicators

Eligibility for government programs (specify, e.g., qualification for federal programs [e.g., WIC, Supplemental Nutrition Assistance Program [refer to state for title of program]], school breakfast/lunch program, food distribution program on U.S. Indian Reservations; state assistance programs, such as emergency food assistance programs])

Participation in government programs (specify patient/client or family/caregiver influence)

Eligibility for community programs (specify, e.g., qualification for community programs such as food pantries, meal sites, and meal delivery programs)

Participation in community programs (specify patient/client or family/caregiver influence)

Examples of the measurement methods or data sources for these indicators:
Patient/client report of eligibility/participation, referral information, home evaluation

Typically used with the following domains of nutrition interventions: Nutrition education, nutrition counseling, coordination of nutrition care

Typically used to determine and to monitor and evaluate change in the following nutrition diagnoses: Limited access to food, inadequate or excessive energy intake

Clinical judgment must be used to select indicators and determine the appropriate measurement techniques and reference standards for a given patient population and setting. Once identified, these indicators, measurement techniques, and reference standards should be identified in policies and procedures or other documents for use in patient/client records, quality or performance improvement, or in formal research projects.

Evaluation

Criteria for Evaluation
Comparison to Goal or Reference Standard:
1) Goal (tailored to patient/client needs)
   OR
2) Reference Standard

Patient/Client Example(s)
Example(s) of one or two of the Nutrition Care Indicators (includes sample initial and reassessment documentation for one of the indicators)

Food/Nutrition Program Participation (FH-6.1)

Indicator(s) Selected

Participation in government programs

Criteria for Evaluation

Comparison to Goal or Reference Standard:

1) Goal: Patient/client is not participating in federal school lunch program as parent has not completed required forms.

   OR

2) Reference Standard: No validated standard exists.

Sample Nutrition Assessment and Monitoring and Evaluation Documentation

Initial nutrition assessment with patient/client	The patient/client not participating in federal school lunch program as the required forms are not complete. Will follow-up with family/guardian and monitor change in school lunch program participation at next appointment.
Reassessment after nutrition intervention	Progress toward goal as patient/client's family/guardian has completed school lunch program forms.

Safe Food/Meal Availability (FH-6.2)

Definition
Availability of enough healthful, safe food

Nutrition Assessment and Monitoring and Evaluation
Indicators

Availability of shopping facilities (specify, e.g., access to facilities with a wide variety of healthful food choices)

Procurement of safe food (specify, e.g., financial resources for obtaining food, community gardens, growing own food, hunting and fishing)

Appropriate meal preparation facilities (specify, e.g., access to cooking apparatus and supplies used in
preparation, sanitary conditions and supplies for meal preparation, appropriate temperatures of hot/cold food)

Availability of safe food storage (specify, e.g., refrigerator/freezer, dry storage, designated containers)

Appropriate storage techniques (specify, e.g., appropriate refrigeration/freezer temperatures, canning/
preservation, length of storage, sanitary conditions)

Identification of safe food (specify, e.g., identification of spoilage, expiration dates, identification of foods containing poisons such as specific berries, mushrooms, etc.)

Examples of the measurement methods or data sources for these indicators: Patient/client report overall food availability/food consumed during the week, referral information, home evaluation

Typically used with the following domains of nutrition interventions: Nutrition education, nutrition counseling, coordination of nutrition care

Typically used to determine and to monitor and evaluate change in the following nutrition diagnoses: Limited access to food, intake of unsafe food, inadequate or excessive energy intake

Clinical judgment must be used to select indicators and determine the appropriate measurement techniques and reference standards for a given patient population and setting. Once identified, these indicators, measurement techniques, and reference standards should be identified in policies and procedures or other documents for use in patient/client records, quality or performance improvement, or in formal research projects.

Evaluation

Criteria for Evaluation
Comparison to Goal or Reference Standard:
1) Goal (tailored to patient/client needs)
OR
2) Reference Standard

Safe Food/Meal Availability (FH-6.2)

Patient/Client Example(s)

Example(s) of one or two of the Nutrition Care Indicators (includes sample initial and reassessment documentation for one of the indicators)

Indicator(s) Selected

Availability of meal preparation facilities

Criteria for Evaluation

Comparison to Goal or Reference Standard:

1. Goal: Patient/client has no access to meal preparation facilities when extensive access to meal preparation facilities is the goal.
   OR
2. Reference Standard: No validated standard exists.

Sample Nutrition Assessment and Monitoring and Evaluation Documentation

Initial nutrition assessment with patient/client	The patient/client has no access to meal preparation facilities. Will monitor change in access at next appointment after coordination of nutrition care with social work.
Reassessment after nutrition intervention	Substantial progress toward goal as patient/client has consistent access to meal preparation facility with repair of stove.

Updated: 2013 Edition

Safe Water Availability (FH-6.3)

Definition
Availability of potable water

Nutrition Assessment and Monitoring and Evaluation
Indicators
Availability of potable water (specify, e.g., functioning well, access to treated public water supply)

Appropriate water decontamination (specify, e.g., awareness of and compliance with public health warnings, use of strategies such as boiling, chemical, filtration treatment)

Examples of the measurement methods or data sources for these indicators:
Patient/client report of water availability and/or decontamination strategies, referral information, home evaluation

Typically used with the following domains of nutrition interventions: Nutrition education, nutrition counseling, coordination of nutrition care

Typically used to determine and to monitor and evaluate change in the following nutrition diagnoses:
Inadequate fluid intake, intake of unsafe food

Clinical judgment must be used to select indicators and determine the appropriate measurement techniques and reference standards for a given patient population and setting. Once identified, these indicators, measurement techniques, and reference standards should be identified in policies and procedures or other documents for use in patient/client records, quality or performance improvement, or in formal research projects.

Evaluation

Criteria for Evaluation
Comparison to Goal or Reference Standard:
1) Goal (tailored to patient/client needs)
    OR
2) Reference Standard

Patient/Client Example(s)
Example(s) of one or two of the Nutrition Care Indicators (includes sample initial and reassessment documentation for one of the indicators)

Indicator(s) Selected
Appropriate water decontamination

Safe Water Availability (FH-6.3)

Criteria for Evaluation

Comparison to Goal or Reference Standard:

1) Goal: Patient/client has limited awareness and no compliance with water decontamination recommendations when extensive awareness and compliance with the decontamination guidelines is the goal.

   OR

2) Reference Standard: No validated standard exists.

Sample Nutrition Assessment and Monitoring and Evaluation Documentation

Initial nutrition assessment with patient/client	The patient/client has limited awareness and no compliance with water decontamination recommendations (e.g., community has a boil water alert for water used for drinking and cooking) when extensive awareness and compliance with the decontamination guidelines is the goal. Will monitor change in compliance at next appointment.
Reassessment after nutrition intervention	Substantial progress toward goal as patient/client is complying with water decontamination guidelines.

Food/Nutrition-Related Supplies Availability (FH-6.4)

Definition
Access to necessary food/nutrition-related supplies

Nutrition Assessment and Monitoring and Evaluation

Indicators

Access to food/nutrition-related supplies (specify, e.g., glucose monitor, monitoring strips, lancets, pedometer, PN/EN supplies, thickeners, blood pressure-related devices)

Access to assistive eating devices (equipment or utensils), specify, e.g., modified utensils, plates, bowls, gavage feeding supplies)

Access to assistive food preparation devices (specify, e.g., modified utensils for food preparation, electric can openers, rocking knives, one-handed devices)

Examples of the measurement methods or data sources for these indicators:
Patient/client report, referral information, home evaluation

Typically used with the following domains of nutrition interventions: Nutrition education, nutrition counseling, coordination of nutrition care

Typically used to determine and to monitor and evaluate change in the following nutrition diagnoses: Inability to manage self-care, inadequate oral intake, self-feeding difficulty, limited adherence to nutrition-related recommendations

Clinical judgment must be used to select indicators and determine the appropriate measurement techniques and reference standards for a given patient population and setting. Once identified, these indicators, measurement techniques, and reference standards should be identified in policies and procedures or other documents for use in patient/client records, quality or performance improvement, or in formal research projects.

Evaluation

Criteria for Evaluation
Comparison to Goal or Reference Standard:
1) Goal (tailored to patient/client needs)
   OR
2) Reference Standard

Patient/Client Example(s)
Example(s) of one or two of the Nutrition Care Indicators (includes sample initial and reassessment documentation for one of the indicators)

Indicator(s) Selected
Access to food/nutrition-related supplies

Food/Nutrition-Related Supplies Availability (FH-6.4)

Criteria for Evaluation

Comparison to Goal or Reference Standard:

    1) Goal: Patient/client has limited access to a sufficient quantity of glucose monitoring strips when extensive access is the goal.

       OR

    2) Reference Standard: No validated standard exists.

Sample Nutrition Assessment and Monitoring and Evaluation Documentation

Initial nutrition assessment with patient/client	The patient/client has limited access to a sufficient quantity of glucose monitoring strips. Will monitor change in access to glucose monitoring strips at next appointment.
Reassessment after nutrition intervention	Some progress toward goal as patient/client has moderate access to a sufficient supply of glucose monitoring strips.

Breastfeeding (FH-7.1)

Definition

Degree to which breastfeeding plans and experience meet nutritional and other needs of the infant and mother

Nutrition Assessment and Monitoring and Evaluation

Indicators

Initiation of breastfeeding
* Breastfeeding attempts (number)

Duration of breastfeeding (specify, e.g., weeks, months, years)

Exclusive breastfeeding (yes/no)

Breastfeeding problems
* Evaluation of latch (correct/incorrect)
* Evaluation of mother's nipples (not irritated/irritated)
* Evaluation of sucking (minutes rhythmic sucking per feeding)
* Presence of breastmilk* in baby's mouth when unlatched from breast (yes/no)
* Evaluation of mother's breasts (specify, e.g., full/firm prior to feeding, soft after feeding)
* Mother's evaluation of baby's satisfaction after feeding (specify, e.g., still hungry/satisfied)
* Other (specify)

> Note: Infant/child growth can be found on the Body Composition/Growth/Weight History reference sheet.
>
> Breastfeeding self-efficacy and intention to breastfeed can be found on the Beliefs and Attitudes reference sheet.
>
> *If a synonym for the term "breastmilk" is helpful or needed, an approved alternate is "human milk."

Examples of the measurement methods or data sources for this indicator: Patient/client report, practitioner observation of breastfeeding, self-monitoring records, infant weight trends

Typically used to determine and monitor and evaluate change in the following domains of nutrition interventions: Nutrition education, nutrition counseling, coordination of nutrition care

Typically used to determine and to monitor and evaluate change in the following nutrition diagnoses: Maternal breastfeeding difficulty, food- and nutrition-related knowledge deficit, unsupported beliefs/attitudes about food- or nutrition-related topics, involuntary weight loss, inadequate fluid intake

Clinical judgment must be used to select indicators and determine the appropriate measurement techniques and reference standards for a given patient population and setting. Once identified, these indicators, measurement techniques, and reference standards should be identified in policies and procedures or other documents for use in patient/client records, quality or performance improvement, or in formal research projects.

Breastfeeding (FH-7.1)

Evaluation

Criteria for Evaluation
Comparison to Goal or Reference Standard:
1) Goal (tailored to patient/client's needs)
   OR
2) Reference Standard

Patient/Client Example(s)
Example(s) of one or two of the Nutrition Care Indicators (includes sample initial and reassessment documentation for one of the indicators)

Indicator(s) Selected
Initiation of breastfeeding

Criteria for Evaluation
Comparison to Goal or Reference Standard:
1) Goal: Patient/client currently fears her breastmilk* supply is not adequate and worries about how she will manage when she returns to work in four weeks. Goal is for mother to breastfeed for six months.
   OR
2) Reference Standard: No validated standard exists.

Sample Nutrition Assessment and Monitoring and Evaluation Documentation

Initial encounter with patient/client	Postpartum patient/client states she is planning to use a combination of formula and breastfeeding and start solids at 3 months. Will educate and refer to lactation support group.
Reassessment after nutrition intervention	Patient/client reports she has exclusively breast fed for three months and plans to delay introduction of solids. Will reinforce and educate. Continue to monitor.

If a synonym for the term "breastmilk" is helpful or needed, an approved alternate is "human milk."

Updated: 2013 Edition

Nutrition-Related Activities of Daily Living and Instrumental Activities of Daily Living (FH-7.2)

Definition

Level of cognitive and physical ability to perform nutrition-related activities of daily living and instrumental activities of daily living by older and/or disabled persons

Nutrition Assessment and Monitoring and Evaluation

Indicators

Physical ability to complete tasks for meal preparation (plan meals, shop for meals, finances, meal preparation) (yes/no)

Physical ability to self-feed (yes/no)

Ability to position self in relation to plate (within 12 to 18 inches (30-45 cm) from mouth to plate) (yes/no)

Receives assistance with intake (yes/no)

Ability to use adaptive eating devices (those that have been deemed necessary and that improve self-feeding skills) (yes/no)

Cognitive ability to complete tasks for meal preparation (planning meals, shopping for meals, finances, meal preparation) (yes/no)

Remembers to eat (yes/no)

Recalls eating (yes/no)

Mini Mental State Examination Score (score)

Nutrition-related activities of daily living (ADL) score (score)

Nutrition-related instrumental activities of daily living (IADL) score (score)

> Note: Sufficient intake of food can be found on the Food Intake reference sheet.
>
> Sufficient intake of fluid can be found on the Fluid/Beverage Intake reference sheet.
>
> Food security and ability to maintain sanitation can be found on the Safe Food/Meal Availability reference sheet.
>
> Ability to maintain weight can be found on the Body Composition/Growth/Weight History reference sheet.

Examples of the measurement methods or data sources for these outcome indicators: Self-report, caregiver report, home visit, targeted questionnaires and monitoring devices, ADL and/or IADL measurement tool, congregate meal site attendance records

Typically used with the following domains of nutrition interventions: Coordination of nutrition care

Typically used to determine and to monitor and evaluate change in the following nutrition diagnoses: Inability to manage self-care, impaired ability to prepare foods/meals

Nutrition-Related Activities of Daily Living and Instrumental Activities of Daily Living (FH-7.2)

Clinical judgment must be used to select indicators and determine the appropriate measurement techniques and reference standards for a given patient population and setting. Once identified, these indicators, measurement techniques, and reference standards should be identified in policies and procedures or other documents for use in patient/client records, quality or performance improvement, or in formal research projects.

Evaluation

Criteria for Evaluation

Comparison to Goal or Reference Standard:
1) Goal (tailored to patient/client's needs)
   OR
2) Reference Standard

Patient/Client Example(s)

Example(s) of one or two of the Nutrition Care Indicators (includes sample initial and reassessment documentation for one of the indicators)

Indicator(s) Selected

Nutrition-related instrumental activities of daily living (IADL) score

Criteria for Evaluation

Comparison to Goal or Reference Standard:
1) Goal: Patient/client with decreased food intake due to an inability to drive, no close relatives living in the vicinity, and difficulty in performing meal preparation tasks due to weakness.
   OR
2) Reference Standard: No validated standard exists.

Sample Nutrition Assessment and Monitoring and Evaluation Documentation

Initial encounter with patient/client	Patient/client with inadequate food intake due to inability to drive, no close relative living in vicinity, subsequent weight loss and difficulties in performing ADLs and IADLs due to weakness. Patient/client is to use new strategies and community resources to facilitate attendance at senior center congregate meals 5 times per week, use of community-provided transportation offered to grocery store 1 x per week, and attendance in strength training at senior center.
Reassessment after nutrition intervention	Significant progress in nutrition-related activities of daily living. Patient/client able to attend senior center for meals and strength training 3 times this week. Goal is 5 times. Will continue to assess at next encounter. Patient/client going to grocery store 1 x per week.

Updated: 2013 Edition

ASSESSMENT/MON & EVAL

Physical Activity (FH-7.3)

Definition
Level of physical activity and/or amount of exercise performed

Nutrition Assessment and Monitoring and Evaluation
Indicators
Physical activity history (e.g., activities, preferences, attitudes)

Consistency (yes/no)

Frequency (number times/week)

Duration (number minutes/session, number of total minutes/day)

Intensity (e.g., talk test, Borg Rating of Perceived Exertion, % of predetermined max heart rate)

Type of physical activity (e.g., cardiovascular, muscular strength/endurance, flexibility; lifestyle, programmed)

Strength (e.g., grip strength or other muscle strength measure)

TV/screen time (minutes/day)

Other sedentary activity time (e.g., commuting; sitting at desk, in meetings, at sporting or arts events) (minutes/day)

Involuntary physical movement (present/absent)

NEAT (Non-exercise activity thermogensis) (present/absent, level)

Examples of the measurement methods or data sources for these outcome indicators: History interview/questionnaire, physical activity log, step counter, accelerometer, attendance at strength training, balance training (for older adults), and/or aerobic classes, caretaker records, medical record

Typically used with the following domains of nutrition interventions: Nutrition education, nutrition counseling

Typically used to determine and to monitor and evaluate change in the following nutrition diagnoses: Physical inactivity, excessive exercise, underweight, over-weight/obesity, unintended weight loss or weight gain

Clinical judgment must be used to select indicators and determine the appropriate measurement techniques and reference standards for a given patient population and setting. Once identified, these indicators, measurement techniques, and reference standards should be identified in policies and procedures or other documents for use in patient/client records, quality or performance improvement, or in formal research projects.

Evaluation

Criteria for Evaluation
Comparison to Goal or Reference Standard:
1) Goal (tailored to patient/client's needs)
   OR
2) Reference Standard

Physical Activity (FH-7.3)

Patient/Client Example(s)

Example(s) of one or two of the Nutrition Care Indicators (includes sample initial and reassessment documentation for one of the indicators)

Indicator(s) Selected

Consistency and duration

Criteria for Evaluation

Comparison to Goal or Reference Standard:

1) Goal: Patient/client typically walks approximately 10 minutes, twice per week. Patient/client goal is to walk approximately 15 minutes, 5 days per week.

OR

2) Reference Standard: Patient/client's typical 10-minute walk, twice a week is well below the recommended at least 30 minutes of moderate-intensity physical activity (in bouts 10 minutes or longer), 5 days per week or at least 20 minutes of vigorous intensity physical activity (in bouts 10 minutes or longer), 3 days per week (ACSM/AHA Physical Activity Guidelines for Public Health for adults and seniors)

Sample Nutrition Assessment and Monitoring and Evaluation Documentation

Initial encounter with patient/client	Based on exercise log, patient/client doing moderate-intensity physical activities 30 minutes/day, 2 days/week. Goal is to do at least 30 minutes/day (in bouts 10 minutes or longer), moderate-intensity activities, 5 or more days/wk. Will monitor physical activity level at next appointment.
Reassessment after nutrition intervention	Significant progress toward goal of exercising at 30 minutes/day, moderate-intensity activities, 5 or more days/wk. Patient/client reports doing moderate-intensity activities 30 minutes per day, 4 days/week.

Updated: 2011 Edition

ASSESSMENT/MON & EVAL

Factors Affecting Access to Physical Activity (FH-7.4)

Definition

Factors influencing access to physical activity opportunities and physical activity participation

Nutrition Assessment and Monitoring and Evaluation

Indicators

Neighborhood safety (the patient/client's perception of crime and traffic, presence of gangs, witness to physical attacks, presence of community members walking or playing outside and feeling it is safe to walk outside. Patient/client rate on a scale of 1 to 10, 1=Unsafe, 10=Safe)

Walkability of neighborhood (the patient/client's perception on his/her ability to walk in a neighborhood related to street connectivity, road type, dwelling density, and land use attributes (i.e., residential, commercial, institutional or industrial land use). Patient/client rate on a scale of 1 to 10, 1=Not walkable, 10=Very walkable)

Proximity to parks/green space (the patient/client's perception of the distance from the patient's home/workplace to the nearest park/green space. Patient/client rate on a scale of 1 to 10, 1=Large distance to nearest park/green space, 10=Small distance to nearest park/green space)

Access to physical activity facilities/programs (the patient/client's perception of the availability of physical activity facilities/programs in the patient's environment. Patient/client rate on a scale of 1 to 10, 1=No availability of facilities/programs, 10=Excellent availability of facilities/programs)

> Note: Physical disability, mobility and socioeconomic factors affecting physical activity can be documented in the in Personal data (CH-1.1) and Social history (CH-3.1).

Examples of the measurement methods or data sources for these outcome indicators: Patient perception, neighborhood crime statistics, neighborhood traffic statistics, geographic information systems data to map a neighborhood, availability of retail establishments within walking distance

Typically used with the following domains of nutrition interventions: Nutrition education, nutrition counseling and coordination of care

Typically used to determine and to monitor and evaluate change in the following nutrition diagnoses: overweight/obesity, physical inactivity, not ready for diet/lifestyle change

Clinical judgment must be used to select indicators and determine the appropriate measurement techniques and reference standards for a given patient population and setting. Once identified, these indicators, measurement techniques, and reference standards should be identified in policies and procedures or other documents for use in patient/client records, quality or performance improvement, or in formal research projects.

ASSESSMENT/MON & EVAL

Factors Affecting Access to Physical Activity (FH-7.4)

Evaluation

Criteria for Evaluation
Comparison to Goal or Reference Standard:
1) Goal (tailored to patient/client's needs)
   OR
2) Reference Standard

Patient/Client Example(s)
Example(s) of one or two of the Nutrition Care Indicators (includes sample initial and reassessment documentation for one of the indicators)

Indicator(s) Selected
Neighborhood safety

Criteria for Evaluation
Comparison to Goal or Reference Standard:
1) Goal: Patient rated neighborhood as unsafe when increased physical activity is a goal.
   OR
2) Reference Standard:

Sample Nutrition Assessment and Monitoring and Evaluation Documentation

Initial encounter with patient/client	Patient perceives that the neighborhood is unsafe (self-perception rating of a 2) for an individual to engage in outdoor exercise alone because of environmental factors (e.g. crime, traffic, gang presence, witness to physical attack) and has limited compliance with increasing physical activity.
Reassessment after nutrition intervention	Patient has joined a neighborhood outdoor exercise group and now rates neighborhood safety as a 7 and has increasing compliance with regular physical activity.

Created: 2013 Edition

Nutrition Quality of Life* (FH-8.1)

Definition
Extent to which the Nutrition Care Process impacts a patient/client's physical, mental, and social well-being related to food and nutrition

Nutrition Assessment and Monitoring and Evaluation
Indicators
Nutrition quality of life responses

> Note: A nutrition quality of life instrument has been developed and is being validated (Barr JT, et al 2003). Focused questioning around the six indicators using the 50 NQOL statements is recommended.

Examples of the measurement methods or data sources for these outcome indicators: Nutrition Quality of Life measurement tool, other quality of life tools

Typically used with the following domains of nutrition interventions: Food and/or nutrient delivery, supplements, nutrition education, nutrition counseling, coordination of nutrition care

Typically used to determine and to monitor and evaluate change in the following nutrition diagnoses: Poor nutrition quality of life, inadequate or excessive energy or macronutrient intake, underweight, unintended weight loss, overweight/obesity, unintended weight gain, disordered eating pattern, inability to manage self-care, swallowing difficulty, chewing difficulty, self-feeding difficulty, altered GI function, limited access to food and/or water

Clinical judgment must be used to select indicators and determine the appropriate measurement techniques and reference standards for a given patient population and setting. Once identified, these indicators, measurement techniques, and reference standards should be identified in policies and procedures or other documents for use in patient/client records, quality or performance improvement, or in formal research projects.

Evaluation

Criteria for Evaluation
Comparison to Goal or Reference Standard:
1) Goal (tailored to patient/client's needs)
   OR
2) Reference Standard

Patient/Client Example(s)
Example(s) of one or two of the Nutrition Care Indicators (includes sample initial and reassessment documentation for one of the indicators)

Indicator(s) Selected
Nutrition quality of life score

* This nutrition indicator is included to encourage further research.

Nutrition Quality of Life* (FH-8.1)

Criteria for Evaluation

Comparison to Goal or Reference Standard:

1) Goal: Patient/client with chronic renal disease currently reports poor nutrition quality of life, especially decreased walking ability (physical) and limited food choices on renal diet (food impact). The goal of medical nutrition therapy is to educate and coach patient and his family on options and strategies to significantly enhance his nutrition quality of life.

    OR

2. Reference Standard: No validated standard exists.

Sample Nutrition Assessment and Monitoring and Evaluation Documentation

Initial encounter with patient/client	Patient/client with chronic renal disease reports poor nutrition quality of life, particularly in physical and food impact aspects. Patient/client to receive intensive medical nutrition therapy with a goal to improve client's overall nutrition quality of life over a 6-month period. Will monitor nutrition quality of life in 6 months.
Reassessment after nutrition intervention	Some progress toward goal. Patient/client's nutrition quality of life is increased, but further improvement is desired in the physical dimension. Will continue medical nutrition therapy and reassess in 3 months.

* This nutrition indicator is included to encourage further research.

Body Composition/Growth/Weight History (AD-1.1)

Definition
Comparative measures of the body, including fat, muscle, and bone components and growth

Nutrition Assessment and Monitoring and Evaluation
Indicators
Height/length
- Height/length (in/cm)
- Birth length (in/cm)
- Pre-amputation height (in/cm)
- Estimated height
  - Knee height (cm)
  - Arm span (in/cm)

Weight
- Weight (lb, oz, kg, g)
- Measured
- Stated
- Usual body weight (UBW) (lb/kg)
- UBW percentage (%)
- Birth weight
- Dosing weight (lb, oz, kg, g)
- Dry weight (lb, oz, kg, g)

Frame size
- Frame size (small/medium/large)

Weight change
- Weight change (specify lb, kg, oz, g, %)
  Specify time frame: _____
- Intent (intentional/unintentional)
- Weight change, interdialytic (% dry weight)
- Weight change, gestational (lb, oz, kg, g)
  Specify time frame: _____

Body mass index
- Body mass index (BMI) (kg/m^2)
- BMI prime (actual BMI/upper limit BMI)

Growth pattern indices/percentile ranks
- Corrected age for prematurity
- BMI percentile/age (percentile rank)
- Head circumference (cm or in)
- Head circumference-for-age (percentile rank)
- Length/stature-for-age (percentile rank)
- Weight-for-length/stature (percentile rank)
- Weight-for-age (percentile rank)

Body Composition/Growth/Weight History (AD-1.1)

Indicators, cont'd

Body compartment estimates

- Body fat percentage (%)
- Body surface area (m²)
- Bone age (years)
- Bone mineral density (units)
- Mid-arm muscle circumference (percentile rank)
- Triceps skin fold (percentile rank)
- Waist circumference (in or cm)
- Waist hip ratio (ratio)

Examples of the measurement methods or data sources for these outcome indicators: Referring health care provider or agency, direct measurement, patient/client report, medical record

Typically used with the following domains of nutrition interventions: Food and nutrient delivery, nutrition education, nutrition counseling, coordination of nutrition care

Typically used to determine and monitor and evaluate change in the following nutrition diagnoses: Excessive or inadequate intake of energy, fat, protein, carbohydrate, alcohol, and/or mineral intake; underweight, overweight, physical inactivity, excessive exercise

Clinical judgment must be used to select indicators and determine the appropriate measurement techniques and reference standards for a given patient population and setting. Once identified, these indicators, measurement techniques, and reference standards should be identified in policies and procedures or other documents for use in patient/client records, quality or performance improvement, or in formal research projects.

Evaluation

Criteria for Evaluation

Comparison to Goal or Reference Standard:

1) Goal (tailored to patient/client's needs)
   OR
2) Reference Standard

Patient/Client Example(s)

Example(s) of one or two of the Nutrition Care Indicators (includes sample initial and reassessment documentation for one of the indicators)

Indicator(s) Selected

Weight change/day

BMI percentile/age

Body Composition/Growth/Weight History (AD-1.1)

Criteria for Evaluation

Comparison to Goal or Reference Standard:

1) Goal: The infant is only gaining, on average, 10 grams per day compared with a goal weight gain of 20 to 30 grams per day.

   OR

2) Reference Standard: Child's (> age 3 years) BMI percentile/age per growth curves has crossed 2 percentile channels from 50% to 10% in last 6 months.

Sample Nutrition Assessment and Monitoring and Evaluation Documentation

Initial nutrition assessment with patient/client	Child's BMI percentile/age per growth curves has crossed 2 percentile channels from 50% to 10% in last 6 months. Will monitor BMI percentile/age at next encounter.
Reassessment after nutrition intervention	Child's BMI percentile/age per growth curves is unchanged from baseline measure.

Acid Base Balance (BD-1.1)

Definition

Balance between acids and bases in the body fluids. The pH (hydrogen ion concentration) of the arterial blood provides an index for the total body acid-base balance (1).

Nutrition Assessment

Indicators

pH (number)

Arterial bicarbonate, HCO3 (mmol/L)

Partial pressure of carbon dioxide in arterial blood, $PaCO_2$ (mmHg)

Partial pressure of oxygen in arterial blood, PaO_2 (mmHg)

Venous pH (number)

Venous bicarbonate, CO_2 (mmol/L)

Note: Sodium and chloride can be found on the Electrolyte and Renal Profile reference sheet

Examples of the measurement methods or data sources for these indicators:
Biochemical measurement, laboratory report

Typically used with the following domains of nutrition interventions: Food and/or nutrient delivery, coordination of nutrition care

Typically used to determine and to monitor and evaluate change in the following nutrition diagnoses: Altered nutrition-related laboratory values

Clinical judgment must be used to select indicators and determine the appropriate measurement techniques and reference standards for a given patient population and setting. Once identified, these indicators, measurement techniques, and reference standards should be identified in policies and procedures or other documents for use in patient/client records, quality or performance improvement, or in formal research projects.

Evaluation

Criteria for Evaluation

Comparison to Goal or Reference Standard:
1) Goal (tailored to patient/client's needs)
   OR
2) Reference Standard

Patient/Client Example

Example(s) of one or two of the Nutrition Care Indicators (includes sample initial and reassessment documentation for one of the indicators)

Indicator(s) Selected

pH, serum (number)

Acid Base Balance (BD-1.1)

Criteria for Evaluation

Comparison to Goal or Reference Standard:

1) Goal: Not generally used.

OR

2) Reference Standard: The patient/client pH is 7.48 which is above (above, below, or within expected range) the reference standard (7.35 to 7.45).

Sample nutrition assessment documentation

Initial nutrition assessment with patient/client	Patient/client's pH is 7.48, which is above expected range. Will monitor change in pH at next arterial blood gas.
Reassessment after nutrition intervention	Significant progress toward reference standard. Patient/client's pH is 7.40, within expected range.

Electrolyte and Renal Profile (BD-1.2)

Definition
Laboratory measures associated with electrolyte balance and kidney function

Nutrition Assessment and Monitoring and Evaluation
Indicators

BUN (mg/dL or mmol/L)

Creatinine (mg/dL or μmol/L)

BUN:creatinine ratio (ratio number)

Glomerular filtration rate (mL/min/1.73 m^2)

Sodium (mEq/L or mmol/L)

Chloride (mEq/L or mmol/L)

Potassium (mEq/L or mmol/L)

Magnesium (mEq/L or mmol/L)

Calcium, serum (mg/dL or mmol/L)

Calcium, ionized (mg/dL or mmol/L)

Phosphorus (mg/dL or mmol/L)

Serum osmolality (mOsm/kg or mmol/kg)

Parathyroid hormone (pg/mL or ng/L)

> Note: Bicarbonate can be found on the Acid Base Balance reference sheet.
> Serum albumin can be found on the Protein Profile reference sheet for adjustment of serum calcium.

Examples of the measurement methods or data sources for these indicators:
Biochemical measurement, laboratory report

Typically used with the following domains of nutrition interventions: Food and/or nutrient delivery, coordination of nutrition care

Typically used to determine and to monitor and evaluate change in the following nutrition diagnoses: Excessive or inadequate intake of protein or minerals

Clinical judgment must be used to select indicators and determine the appropriate measurement techniques and reference standards for a given patient population and setting. Once identified, these indicators, measurement techniques, and reference standards should be identified in policies and procedures or other documents for use in patient/client records, quality or performance improvement, or in formal research projects.

Evaluation

Criteria for Evaluation
Comparison to Goal or Reference Standard:
1) Goal (tailored to patient/client's needs)
   OR
2) Reference Standard

Electrolyte and Renal Profile (BD-1.2)

Patient/Client Example
Example(s) of one or two of the Nutrition Care Indicators (includes sample initial and reassessment documentation for one of the indicators)

Indicator(s) Selected
Potassium (mEq/L)

Criteria for Evaluation
Comparison to Goal or Reference Standard:

1) Goal: A goal of serum K+ 3.5 to 5.5 mEq/L in patient/client on medications that block the renin-angiotensin system.
   OR
2) Reference Standard: The patient/client's potassium is 2.9 mEq/L, which is below (above, below, within expected range) the expected range (3.5 to 5.0 mEq/L).

Sample Nutrition Assessment and Monitoring and Evaluation Documentation

Initial nutrition assessment with patient/client	Patient/client's serum potassium is 2.9 mEq/L, which is below the expected range. Will monitor change in potassium at next encounter.
Reassessment after nutrition intervention	Regression from reference standard. Patient/client's potassium is 2.7 mEq/L, below the expected range.

Essential Fatty Acid Profile (BD-1.3)

Definition
Laboratory measures of essential fatty acids

Nutrition Assessment and Monitoring and Evaluation
Indicators
Triene:Tetraene ratio (ratio number)

Examples of the measurement methods or data sources for these indicators:
Biochemical measurement, laboratory report/record

Typically used with the following domains of nutrition interventions: Food and/or nutrient delivery, coordination of nutrition care

Typically used to determine and to monitor and evaluate change in the following nutrition diagnoses: Inadequate intake of fat, parenteral nutrition; less than optimal parenteral nutrition composition or modality; altered nutrition-related laboratory values; impaired nutrient utilization

Clinical judgment must be used to select indicators and determine the appropriate measurement techniques and reference standards for a given patient population and setting. Once identified, these indicators, measurement techniques, and reference standards should be identified in policies and procedures or other documents for use in patient/client records, quality or performance improvement, or in formal research projects.

Evaluation

Criteria for Evaluation
Comparison to Goal or Reference Standard:
1) Goal (tailored to patient/client's needs)
   OR
2) Reference Standard

Patient/Client Example
Example(s) of one or two of the Nutrition Care Indicators (includes sample initial and reassessment documentation for one of the indicators)

Indicator(s) Selected
Triene:Tetraene ratio (ratio number)

Criteria for Evaluation
Comparison to Goal or Reference Standard:
1) Goal: Not generally used.
   OR
2) Reference Standard: The patient/client Triene:Tetraene ratio is 0.45, which is (above, below, or within expected range) above expected range (> 0.2-0.4 essential fatty acid deficiency).

Essential Fatty Acid Profile (BD-1.3)

Sample Nutrition Assessment and Monitoring and Evaluation Documentation

Initial nutrition assessment with patient/client	Patient/client's Triene:Tetraene ratio is 0.45, above the expected range (essential fatty acid deficiency). Will monitor change in Triene:Tetraene ratio at next encounter.
Reassessment after nutrition intervention	Significant progress toward the expect range. Patient/client's Triene:Tetraene ratio is 0.1.

Gastrointestinal Profile (BD-1.4)

Definition
Laboratory measures and medical tests associated with function of the gastrointestinal tract and related organs

Nutrition Assessment and Monitoring and Evaluation
Indicators
Alkaline phosphatase (U/L)

Alanine aminotransferase, ALT (U/L)

Aspartate aminotransferase, AST (U/L)

Gamma glutamyl transferase, GGT (U/L)

Gastric residual volume (mL)

Bilirubin, total (mg/dL or μmol/L)

Ammonia, serum (μg/dL or μmol/L)

Toxicology report, including alcohol (by report)

Prothrombin time, PT (seconds)

Partial thromboplastin time, PTT (seconds)

INR (ratio)

Fecal fat (g/day or g/24 hours)

Amylase (U/L)

Lipase (U/L)

Other digestive enzymes, specify

D-xylose(blood mg/dL; urine % or grams)

Hydrogen breath test (points)

Intestinal biopsy (by report)

Stool culture (by report)

Gastric emptying time (minutes)

Small bowel transit time (minutes, hours)

Abdominal films (by report)

Swallow study (by report)

Examples of the measurement methods or data sources for these indicators: Biochemical measurement, laboratory report

Typically used with the following domains of nutrition interventions: Food and/or nutrient delivery, nutrition education, nutrition counseling

Typically used to determine and to monitor and evaluate change in the following nutrition diagnoses: Altered nutrition-related laboratory values, excess intake of protein or fat

Gastrointestinal Profile (BD-1.4)

Clinical judgment must be used to select indicators and determine the appropriate measurement techniques and reference standards for a given patient population and setting. Once identified, these indicators, measurement techniques, and reference standards should be identified in policies and procedures or other documents for use in patient/client records, quality or performance improvement, or in formal research projects.

Evaluation

Criteria for Evaluation
Comparison to Goal or Reference Standard:
1) Goal (tailored to patient/client's needs)
   OR
2) Reference Standard

Patient/Client Example
Example(s) of one or two of the Nutrition Care Indicators (includes sample initial and reassessment documentation for one of the indicators)

Indicator(s) Selected
Ammonia, serum (µg/dL)

Criteria for Evaluation
Comparison to Goal or Reference Standard:
1) Goal: The patient/client's serum ammonia is 105 µg/dL, which is above the goal (< 75 µg/dL) for this patient/client with end-stage liver disease.
   OR
2) Reference Standard: The patient/client serum ammonia is 85 µg/dL which is above (above, below, or percent of) the expected range (11-35 µg/dL).

Sample Nutrition Assessment and Monitoring and Evaluation Documentation

Initial nutrition assessment with patient/client	Patient/client's serum ammonia is 85 µg/dL, above the expected range. Will monitor change in serum ammonia at next encounter.
Reassessment after nutrition intervention	Significant progress toward expected range. Patient/client's serum ammonia 45 µg/dL.

Updated: 2013 Edition

Glucose/Endocrine Profile (BD-1.5)

Definition

Laboratory measures associated with glycemic control and endocrine findings

Nutrition Assessment and Monitoring and Evaluation

Indicators

Glucose, fasting (mg/dL, mmol/L)

Glucose, casual (mg/dL, mmol/L)

HgbA1c (%, mmol/mol)

Preprandial capillary plasma glucose (mg/dL, mmol/L)

Peak postprandial capillary plasma glucose (mg/dL, mmol/L)

Gluscose tolerance test (mg/dL, mmol/L)

Cortisol level (µg/dL, mmol/L)

IGF-binding protein (ng/mL, mg/L)

Thyroid function tests—TSH, Thyroid stimulating hormone (mIU/L); T4, Thyroxine test (µg/dL); T3, Triiodothyronine (ng/dL, pmol/L)

Pituitary hormone tests-- growth hormone (GH) ng/mL, adrenocorticotropic hormone (ACTH) ng/L, luteinizing hormone (LH) IU/L and follicle-stimulating hormone (FSH) IU/L

Examples of the measurement methods or data sources for these indicators: Biochemical measurement, laboratory report

Typically used with the following domains of nutrition interventions: Food and/or nutrient delivery, nutrition education, nutrition counseling

Typically used to determine and to monitor and evaluate change in the following nutrition diagnoses: Excessive or inadequate intake of carbohydrate, energy; less than optimal intake of types of carbohydrates; or inconsistent carbohydrate intake

Clinical judgment must be used to select indicators and determine the appropriate measurement techniques and reference standards for a given patient population and setting. Once identified, these indicators, measurement techniques, and reference standards should be identified in policies and procedures or other documents for use in patient/client records, quality or performance improvement, or in formal research projects.

Evaluation

Criteria for Evaluation

Comparison to Goal or Reference Standard:

1) Goal (tailored to patient/client's needs)
   OR
2) Reference Standard

Glucose/Endocrine Profile (BD-1.5)

Patient/Client Example
Example(s) of one or two of the Nutrition Care Indicators (includes sample initial and reassessment documentation for one of the indicators)

Indicator(s) Selected
HgbA1c (%, mmol/mol)

Criteria for Evaluation
Comparison to Goal or Reference Standard:
1) Goal: The patient/client's HgbA1c is 7.8% (60 mmol/mol), which is above the expected limit, but is an acceptable goal in a pediatric patient.
   OR
2) Reference Standard: The patient/client's HgbA1c is 11% (97 mmol/mol), which is above (above, below, expected limit or range) the expected limit (< 6%, 42 mmol/mol).

Sample Nutrition Assessment and Monitoring and Evaluation Documentation

Initial nutrition assessment with patient/client	Patient/client's HgbA1c is 9% (75 mmol/mol), which is above the expected limit. Will monitor change in HgbA1c at next encounter.
Reassessment after nutrition intervention	Regression from the expected limit. Patient/client's HgbA1c is 10% (86 mmol/mol).

Updated: 2013 Edition

Inflammatory Profile (BD-1.6)

Definition
Laboratory measures of inflammatory proteins

Nutrition Assessment

Indicators

C-reactive protein, highly sensitive or hs-CRP (mg/L) [cardiovascular disease]

Examples of the measurement methods or data sources for these indicators:
Direct measurement, medical record

Typically used with the following domains of nutrition interventions: Food and/or nutrient delivery

Typically used to determine the following nutrition diagnoses: Increased nutrient need; less than optimal intake of types of fats; excessive physical activity

Clinical judgment must be used to select indicators and determine the appropriate measurement techniques and reference standards for a given patient population and setting. Once identified, these indicators, measurement techniques, and reference standards should be identified in policies and procedures or other documents for use in patient/client records, quality or performance improvement, or in formal research projects.

Evaluation

Criteria for Evaluation

Comparison to Goal or Reference Standard:

1) Goal (tailored to patient/client's needs)
   OR
2) Reference Standard

Patient/Client Example

Example(s) of one or two of the Nutrition Care Indicators (includes sample initial and reassessment documentation for one of the indicators)

Indicator(s) Selected

C-reactive protein (mg/L)

Criteria for Evaluation

Comparison to Goal or Reference Standard:

1) Goal: Not generally used.
   OR
2) Reference Standard: A patient/client has a C-reactive protein level of 4.0 mg/L, which is above (above, below, within expected range) the expected range of 1.0 to 3.0 mg/L.

Sample nutrition assessment documentation

Nutrition assessment with patient/client	Patient/client's C-reactive protein level is 4.0 mg/L, which is above (above, below, within expected range) the expected range of 1.0 to 3.0 mg/L.

Lipid Profile (BD-1.7)

Definition
Laboratory measures associated with lipid disorders

Nutrition Assessment and Monitoring and Evaluation
Indicators
Cholesterol, serum (mg/dL or mmol/L)

Cholesterol, HDL (mg/dL or mmol/L)

Cholesterol, LDL (mg/dL or mmol/L)

Cholesterol, non-HDL (mg/dL or mmol/L)

Total cholesterol:HDL cholesterol (ratio)

LDL:HDL (ratio)

Triglycerides, serum (mg/ dL or mmol/L)

Examples of the measurement methods or data sources for these indicators:
Biochemical measurement, laboratory report, patient/client report

Typically used with the following domains of nutrition interventions: Nutrition education, nutrition counseling

Typically used to determine and to monitor and evaluate change in the following nutrition diagnoses: Excessive or inadequate intake of fat, energy

Clinical judgment must be used to select indicators and determine the appropriate measurement techniques and reference standards for a given patient population and setting. Once identified, these indicators, measurement techniques, and reference standards should be identified in policies and procedures or other documents for use in patient/client records, quality or performance improvement, or in formal research projects.

Evaluation

Criteria for Evaluation
Comparison to Goal or Reference Standard:
1) Goal (tailored to patient/client's needs)
   OR
2) Reference Standard

Patient/Client Example
Example(s) of one or two of the Nutrition Care Indicators (includes sample initial and reassessment documentation for one of the indicators)

Indicator(s) Selected
LDL cholesterol (mg/dL)

Lipid Profile (BD-1.7)

Criteria for Evaluation

Comparison to Goal or Reference Standard:

1) Goal: The patient/client's LDL cholesterol is 200 mg/dL, compared to a goal of < 100 mg/dL. (Note: While reference standards are generally used for laboratory measures, a goal might be used in a special situation such as this example. The patient/client has a familial hypercholesterolemia where a normal reference standard may not be realistic.)
   OR

2) Reference Standard: The patient/client's LDL cholesterol is 159 mg/dL, which is above the expected limit of the NHLBI recommendation of < 100 mg/dL.

Sample Nutrition Assessment and Monitoring and Evaluation Documentation

Initial nutrition assessment with patient/client	The patient/client LDL cholesterol is 159 mg/dL compared to the reference standard (e.g., National Heart, Lung and Blood Institute) recommended level of < 100 mg/dL. Will monitor LDL cholesterol at next encounter.
Reassessment after nutrition intervention	Some progress toward goal/reference standard as patient/client's LDL cholesterol is 145 mg/dL.

Updated: 2013 Edition

Metabolic Rate Profile (BD-1.8)

Definition
Measures associated with or having implications for assessing metabolic rate

Nutrition Assessment and Monitoring and Evaluation
Indicators
Resting metabolic rate, measured (calories, kcal or kJ/day)

Respiratory quotient, measured ($RQ = CO_2$ produced/O_2 consumed)

> *Note: Use of RQ is considered valid if respiratory factors (hyper- or hypoventilation), equipment failure, measurement protocol violations, or operator errors have not occurred.*

Examples of the measurement methods or data sources for these indicators:
Direct measurement (indirect calorimetry), medical record

Typically used with the following domains of nutrition interventions: Food and/or nutrient delivery

Typically used to determine the following nutrition diagnoses: Excessive or inadequate intake of parenteral/enteral nutrition; less than optimal enteral/parenteral nutrition; excessive energy intake; excessive mineral intake; disordered eating pattern; excessive exercise, increased energy expenditure, increased nutrient needs (energy), inadequate protein-energy intake.

Clinical judgment must be used to select indicators and determine the appropriate measurement techniques and reference standards for a given patient population and setting. Once identified, these indicators, measurement techniques, and reference standards should be identified in policies and procedures or other documents for use in patient/client records, quality or performance improvement, or in formal research projects.

Evaluation

Criteria for Evaluation
Comparison to Goal or Reference Standard:
1) Goal (tailored to patient/client's needs)
   OR
2) Reference Standard

Patient/Client Example
Example(s) of one or two of the Nutrition Care Indicators (includes sample initial and reassessment documentation for one of the indicators)

Indicator(s) Selected
Respiratory quotient

Metabolic Rate Profile (BD-1.8)

Criteria for Evaluation
Comparison to Goal or Reference Standard:
1) Goal: Not generally used.
   OR
2) Reference Standard: A patient/client on parenteral nutrition support with an RQ of 1.04, which is above (above, below, within expected range) the expected range (0.7 to 1.0) with no apparent errors in the measurement.

Sample nutrition assessment and/or monitoring and evaluation documentation

Initial nutrition assessment with patient/client	Patient/client's RQ is 1.04, with energy intake from parenteral nutrition 400 kcal (1,670 kJ) higher than measured metabolic rate. No apparent respiratory factors (hyper- or hypoventilation), equipment failure, measurement protocol violations, or operator errors. Will adjust content of parenteral nutrition and re-measure RQ.
Reassessment after nutrition intervention	RQ has dropped to 0.92 with no apparent measurement error. Metabolic rate and calorie/ kcal/kJ intake are matched. Parenteral nutrition has been appropriately adjusted to equal patient's energy requirement.

Mineral Profile (BD-1.9)

Definition
Laboratory measures associated with body mineral status

Nutrition Assessment and Monitoring and Evaluation
Indicators

Copper, serum or plasma (μg/dL or μmol/L)

Iodine, urinary excretion (μg/24hr)

Zinc, serum or plasma (μg/dL or μmol/L)

Boron, serum or plasma (μg/L)

Chromium, serum (ng/mL or nmol/L), urinary (μg/L)

Fluoride, plasma (μmol/L)

Manganese, urinary excretion (μg/L or nmol/L), blood (μg/L or nmol/L), plasma (μg/L or nmol/L)

Molybdenum, serum (ng/mL)

Selenium, serum (μmol/L), urinary excretion (μg/L or μg/day)

> Note: Other measures of body mineral status, such as urinary manganese excretion, are provided to offer complete information in the reference sheet. These are rarely used in practice, but may be warranted in limited circumstances.
>
> Serum calcium, magnesium, phosphorus, and potassium can be found on the Electrolyte and Renal Profile reference sheet.
>
> Serum iron, serum ferritin, and transferrin saturation can be found on the Nutritional Anemia Profile reference sheet.
>
> Thyroid stimulating hormone (↑ TSH as an indicator of excess iodine supplementation) can be found on the Glucose/Endocrine Profile reference sheet.

Examples of the measurement methods or data sources for these indicators:
Biochemical measurement, laboratory record

Typically used with the following domains of nutrition interventions: Food and/or nutrient delivery, nutrition education, nutrition counseling

Typically used to determine and to monitor and evaluate change in the following nutrition diagnoses: Excessive or inadequate intake of minerals, parenteral nutrition

Clinical judgment must be used to select indicators and determine the appropriate measurement techniques and reference standards for a given patient population and setting. Once identified, these indicators, measurement techniques, and reference standards should be identified in policies and procedures or other documents for use in patient/client records, quality or performance improvement, or in formal research projects.

Evaluation

Criteria for Evaluation
Comparison to Goal or Reference Standard:
1) Goal (tailored to patient/client's needs)
   OR
2) Reference Standard

Mineral Profile (BD-1.9)

Patient/Client Example

Example(s) of one or two of the Nutrition Care Indicators (includes sample initial and reassessment documentation for one of the indicators)

Indicator(s) Selected

Zinc, plasma (µg/dL)

Criteria for Evaluation

Comparison to Goal or Reference Standard:

1) Goal: There is no goal generally associated with mineral status.
   OR
2) Reference Standard: The patient/client's plasma zinc is 40 µg/dL, which is below (above, below, within expected range) the expected range (66 to 110 µg/dL) for adults.

Sample Nutrition Assessment and Monitoring and Evaluation Documentation

Initial nutrition assessment with patient/client	Patient/client's plasma zinc is 40 µg/dL, which is below the expected range for adults. Will monitor change in plasma zinc at next encounter.
Reassessment after nutrition intervention	Goal/reference standard achieved as patient/client's plasma zinc is 90 µg/dL.

Updated: 2013 Edition

Nutritional Anemia Profile (BD-1.10)

Definition
Laboratory measures associated with nutritional anemias

Nutrition Assessment and Monitoring and Evaluation
Indicators
Hemoglobin (g/dL g/L or mmol/L)

Hematocrit (% or proportion of one (1))

Mean corpuscular volume, MCV (fL)

RBC folate (ng/mL or nmol/L)

Red cell distribution width, RDW (%)

Serum B12 (pg/mL or pmol/L)

Serum methylmalonic acid, MMA (nmol/L)

Serum folate (ng/mL or nmol/L)

Serum homocysteine (μmol/L)

Serum ferritin (ng/mL or pmol/L)

Serum iron (μg/dL or μmol/L)

Total iron-binding capacity (μg/dL or μmol/L)

Transferrin saturation (%)

Examples of the measurement methods or data sources for these indicators: Biochemical measurement, patient/client laboratory record; national/state/local nutrition monitoring and surveillance data

Typically used with the following domains of nutrition interventions: Food and/or nutrient delivery, nutrition education, nutrition counseling, coordination of nutrition care

Typically used to determine and to monitor and evaluate change in the following nutrition diagnoses: Excessive or inadequate intake of vitamins or minerals (e.g., iron, B12, folate); altered nutrition-related laboratory values; impaired nutrient utilization

Clinical judgment must be used to select indicators and determine the appropriate measurement techniques and reference standards for a given patient population and setting. Once identified, these indicators, measurement techniques, and reference standards should be identified in policies and procedures or other documents for use in patient/client records, quality or performance improvement, or in formal research projects.

Evaluation

Criteria for Evaluation
Comparison to Goal or Reference Standard:
1) Goal (tailored to patient/client's needs)
   OR
2) Reference Standard

Nutritional Anemia Profile (BD-1.10)

Patient/Client Example

Example(s) of one or two of the Nutrition Care Indicators (includes sample initial and reassessment documentation for one of the indicators)

Indicator(s) Selected

Hemoglobin (gm/dL)
Serum ferritin (ng/mL)

Criteria for Evaluation

Comparison to Goal or Reference Standard:

1) Goal: The patient/client's hemoglobin and hematocrit are below the expected limits for adult males, but are within the goal range for a patient/client receiving hemodialysis.

   OR

2) Reference Standard: The patient/client's serum ferritin is 8 ng/mL, which is below (above, below, or within expected range) the expected range for adult females.

Sample Nutrition Assessment and Monitoring and Evaluation Documentation

Initial nutrition assessment with patient/client	Patient/client's serum ferritin is 8 ng/mL, which is below the expected range for adult females. Will monitor change in serum ferritin at next encounter.
Reassessment after nutrition intervention	Patient/client's serum ferritin is 10.9 ng/mL, within the expected range.

Updated: 2013 Edition

Protein Profile (BD-1.11)

Definition
Laboratory measures associated with hepatic and circulating proteins

Nutrition Assessment and Monitoring and Evaluation
Indicators
Albumin (g/dL or g/L)

Prealbumin (mg/dL mg/L)

Transferrin (mg/dL or g/L)

Phenylalanine, plasma (mg/dL or μmol/L)

Tyrosine, plasma (100 μmol/L)

Amino acid, other (by report)

Antibody level, specify

Carbohydrate-deficient transferrin (mg/dL or %)

> Note: Heptatic proteins may be useful when monitoring nutritional status over time in conjunction with other markers/information about nutritional status (e.g., body weight, weight change, nutrient intake).

Examples of the measurement methods or data sources for these indicators:
Biochemical measurement, laboratory report

Typically used with the following domains of nutrition interventions: Food and/or nutrient delivery, nutrition education, nutrition counseling, coordination of nutrition care

Typically used to determine and to monitor and evaluate change in the following nutrition diagnoses: Increased nutrient needs, evident protein-energy malnutrition, inadequate enteral/parenteral nutrition infusion

Clinical judgment must be used to select indicators and determine the appropriate measurement techniques and reference standards for a given patient population and setting. Once identified, these indicators, measurement techniques, and reference standards should be identified in policies and procedures or other documents for use in patient/client records, quality or performance improvement, or in formal research projects.

Evaluation

Criteria for Evaluation
Comparison to Goal or Reference Standard:
1) Goal (tailored to patient/client's needs)
   OR
2) Reference Standard

Patient/Client Example
Example(s) of one or two of the Nutrition Care Indicators (includes sample initial and reassessment documentation for one of the indicators)

Protein Profile (BD-1.11)

Indicator(s) Selected
Prealbumin (mg/dL)

Criteria for Evaluation
Comparison to Goal or Reference Standard:
> 1) Goal: Not generally used.
> OR
> 2) Reference Standard: The patient/client's prealbumin is 7 mg/dL, which is below (above, below, or within the expected range) the expected range (16 to 40 mg/dL) for adults.

Sample Nutrition Assessment and Monitoring and Evaluation Documentation

Initial nutrition assessment with patient/client	Patient/client's prealbumin is 7.0 mg/dL, below the expected range (16 to 40 mg/dL) for adults. Will monitor change in prealbumin at next encounter.
Reassessment after nutrition intervention	Significant progress toward expected range as patient/client's serum prealbumin is 13.0 mg/dL.

Updated: 2013 Edition

Urine Profile (BD-1.12)

Definition
Physical and/or chemical properties of urine

Nutrition Assessment and Monitoring and Evaluation
Indicators
Urine color (by visualization)

Urine osmolality (mOsm/kg H_2O)

Urine specific gravity (number)

Urine tests (e.g., calcium mg/day and/or presence/absence of ketones, sugar, protein, microalbumin)

Urine volume (mL/24 hours; however, in certain populations, e.g., infants, this indicator may be reported in number of wet diapers/day)

Examples of the measurement methods or data sources for these indicators:
Observation, biochemical measurement, laboratory report, patient/client report

Typically used with the following domains of nutrition interventions: Food and/or nutrient delivery, coordination of nutrition care

Typically used to determine and to monitor and evaluate change in the following nutrition diagnoses:
Inadequate or excessive fluid intake; inadequate or excessive enteral/parenteral nutrition infusion

Clinical judgment must be used to select indicators and determine the appropriate measurement techniques and reference standards for a given patient population and setting. Once identified, these indicators, measurement techniques, and reference standards should be identified in policies and procedures or other documents for use in patient/client records, quality or performance improvement, or in formal research projects.

Evaluation

Criteria for Evaluation
Comparison to Goal or Reference Standard:
1) Goal (tailored to patient/client's needs)
   OR
2) Reference Standard

Patient/Client Example
Example(s) of one or two of the Nutrition Care Indicators (includes sample initial and reassessment documentation for one of the indicators)

Indicator(s) Selected
Urine specific gravity

Urine Profile (BD-1.12)

Criteria for Evaluation

Comparison to Goal or Reference Standard:

1) Goal: Not generally used for this indicator.

   OR

2) Reference Standard: The patient/client's urine specific gravity is 1.050, which is above (above, below, within expected range) the expected range (1.003 to 1.030).

Sample Nutrition Assessment and Monitoring and Evaluation Documentation

Initial nutrition assessment with patient/client	Patient/client's urine specific gravity is 1.050, which is above the expected range. Will monitor change in urine specific gravity at next encounter.
Reassessment after nutrition intervention	Significant progress toward goal, patient/client's urine specific gravity is 1.035, which is within the expected range.

Updated: 2013 Edition

Vitamin Profile (BD-1.13)

Definition

Laboratory measures associated with body vitamin status

Nutrition Assessment and Monitoring and Evaluation

Indicators

Vitamin A, serum or plasma retinol (µg/dL or µmol/L)

Vitamin C, plasma or serum (mg/dL or µmol/L)

Vitamin D, 25-hydroxy (ng/mL or nmol/L)

Vitamin E, plasma alpha-tocopherol (mg/dL or µmol/L)

Thiamin, activity coefficient for erythrocyte transketolase activity (µg/mL/hr)

Riboflavin, activity coefficient for erythrocyte glutathione reductase activity (IU/g hemoglobin)

Niacin, urinary N'methyl-nicotinamide concentration (µmol/day)

Vitamin B6, plasma or serum pyridoxal 5'phosphate concentration (ng/mL or nmol/L)

Pantothenic acid, urinary pantothenate excretion (mg/day), plasma (ng/mL or nmol/L)

Biotin, urinary 3-hydroxyisovaleric acid excretion (mmol/mmol creatinine) or lymphocyte propionyl-CoA carboxylase in pregnancy [pmol/(min × mg)], serum (ng/mL or nmol/L)

> Note: Other measures of body vitamin status, such as urinary pantothenate excretion, are provided to offer complete information in the reference sheet. These are rarely used in practice, but may be warranted in limited circumstances.
>
> Measures for folate and Vitamin B12 can be found on the Nutritional Anemia Profile reference sheet.
>
> Measures related to Vitamin K (PT, PTT, INR) can be found on the GI Profile reference sheet.
>
> A test for Choline is not available. According to the DRIs, it should be evaluated in light of serum alanine amino transferase (ALT) levels which can be found on the GI Profile (BD-1.4).

Examples of the measurement methods or data sources for these indicators: Biochemical measurement, patient/client record

Typically used with the following domains of nutrition interventions: Food and/or nutrient delivery, coordination of nutrition care

Typically used to determine and to monitor and evaluate change in the following nutrition diagnoses: Excessive or inadequate intake of vitamins

Clinical judgment must be used to select indicators and determine the appropriate measurement techniques and reference standards for a given patient population and setting. Once identified, these indicators, measurement techniques, and reference standards should be identified in policies and procedures or other documents for use in patient/client records, quality or performance improvement, or in formal research projects.

Vitamin Profile (BD-1.13)

Evaluation

Criteria for Evaluation

Comparison to Goal or Reference Standard:
1) Goal (tailored to patient/client's needs)
     OR
2) Reference Standard

Patient/Client Example

Example(s) of one or two of the Nutrition Care Indicators (includes sample initial and reassessment documentation for one of the indicators)

Indicator(s) Selected:

Vitamin A, serum retinol (μg/dL)

Criteria for Evaluation

Comparison to Goal or Reference Standard:
1) Goal: Not generally used for this indicator.
     OR
2) Reference Standard: The patient/client's serum retinol is 95 μg/dL which is above (above, below, within expected range) the expected range (10 to 60 μg/dL).

Sample Nutrition Assessment and Monitoring and Evaluation Documentation

Initial nutrition assessment with patient/client	Patient/client's serum retinol is 95 μg/dL, which is above the expected range. Will monitor change in serum retinol at next encounter, along with vitamin A and beta- carotene intake.
Reassessment after nutrition intervention	Significant progress toward expected range. Patient/client's retinol is 70 μg/dL.

Updated: 2013 Edition

Nutrition-Focused Physical Findings (PD-1.1)

Definition

Nutrition-related physical characteristics associated with pathophysiological states derived from a nutrition-focused physical exam, interview, or the medical record

Nutrition Assessment and Monitoring and Evaluation

Indicators (Note: Presence or absence unless otherwise specified)

- Overall appearance
  - Body positioning, e.g., muscle contractures
  - Body habitus, specify
  - Cushingoid appearance
  - Amputations, specify
  - Ability to communicate
  - Affect, specify
  - Tanner stage, specify
  - Other
- Body language (note: varies by culture), specify
- Cardiovascular-pulmonary system
  - edema, pulmonary; crackles or rales
  - shortness of breath
- Extremities, muscles and bones
  - bones, specify, obvious prominence, fragility, widening at ends
  - change in how clothes fit, specify
  - edema, peripheral, specify
  - fat, subcutaneous, specify loss or excess
  - fatigue
  - feeling cold all of the time
  - hands/feet, specify, cyanosis, tingling and numbness• joint mobility, wrist/digit/arm/knee/hip movement
  - muscle mass, specify
  - muscle soreness or weakness
  - joint, arthralgia, effusions
  - nails, nail beds, specify, blue, clubbing, pale, other
  - Russell's sign
- Digestive system (mouth to rectum):
  - belching, excessive
  - cheilosis
  - dry mucus membranes, xerostomia
  - feeling of food "stuck" in throat
  - gingivitis
  - heartburn
  - hoarse or wet voice
  - ketone smell on breath, halitosis
  - lesions, oral or esophageal
  - lips, specify (dry or cracked, poor closure, drooling)
  - malformations, oral, e.g., cleft palate or other
  - mastication, altered, specify
  - mucosal edema
  - parotid glands, swollen
  - polydipsia
  - pouching
  - stomatitis
  - swallow function, compromised or painful
  - suck, swallow, breath coordination (infants)
  - taste alterations, specify
  - teeth, specify (edentulous, partially or completely)
  - tongue, specify, bright red, magenta, dry cracked, glossitis, impaired movement, frenulum abnormality
  - abdominal distension, bloating, cramping, pain

Nutrition-Focused Physical Findings (PD-1.1)

- appetite, specify
- ascites
- bowel function, including flatus, specify, e.g., type, frequency, volume
- bowel sounds, specify, normal, hyperactive, hypoactive
- epigastric pain
- nausea
- satiety, specify
- vomiting

- Head and eyes

  Eyes:
  - bitot's spots
  - night blindness
  - sclera, jaundiced
  - sunken eyes
  - vision, specify
  - xerophthalmia

  Head:
  - fontanelle, bulging or sunken
  - hair, specify, brittle, lifeless, coiled, loss
  - headache
  - lanugo hair formation
  - nasal mucosa, dry
  - olfactory sense, altered, specify
  - temporal wasting

- Nerves and cognition
  - confusion, loss of concentration
  - cranial nerve evaluation, specify
  - dizziness
  - motor, gait disturbance
  - neurological changes, other, specify
  - vibratory and position sense, specify

- Skin
  - acanthanosis nigricans
  - calcinosis
  - changes consistent with nutrient deficiency/excess, specify
  - dermatitis
  - dry, scaly
  - ecchymosis
  - erythema, scaling and peeling
  - fistula output, specify volume
  - follicular hyperkeratosis
  - integrity, turgor, specify
  - jaundice
  - perifolicular hemorrhages
  - petechiae
  - pressure ulcers, specify location and stage
  - pruritis
  - seborrheic dermatitis
  - wound healing, specify
  - xanthomas

- Vital signs
  - blood pressure (mmHg)
  - heart rate (beats/min)
  - respiratory rate (breaths/min)
  - temperature (degrees)

Examples of the measurement methods or data sources for these indicators: Direct observation, patient/client report, medical record

Typically used with the following domains of nutrition interventions: Food and nutrient delivery, nutrition education, nutrition counseling, coordination of care

Nutrition-Focused Physical Findings (PD-1.1)

Typically used to determine and to monitor and evaluate change in the following nutrition diagnoses: Excessive or inadequate intake of sodium, vitamins/minerals, fluid, parenteral/enteral nutrition; overweight/obesity, underweight, unintended weight loss

Clinical judgment must be used to select indicators and determine the appropriate measurement techniques and reference standards for a given patient population and setting. Once identified, these indicators, measurement techniques, and reference standards should be identified in policies and procedures or other documents for use in patient/client records, quality or performance improvement, or in formal research projects.

Evaluation

Criteria for Evaluation
Comparison to Goal or Reference Standard:
1) Goal (tailored to patient/client's needs)
   OR
2) Reference Standard

Patient/Client Example
Example(s) of one or two of the Nutrition Care Indicators (includes sample initial and reassessment documentation for one of the indicators)

Indicator(s) Selected
Blood pressure (mmHg)

Criteria for Evaluation
Comparison to Goal or Reference Standard:
1) Goal: The patient/client has reduced blood pressure to goal of 135/85 mmHg with weight loss.
   OR
2) Reference Standard: The patient/client's blood pressure is 150/90 mmHg, which is above (above, below) the expected limit (<120/80 mmHg) and consistent with Stage I Hypertension.

Sample Nutrition Assessment and Monitoring and Evaluation Documentation

Initial nutrition assessment with patient/client	Patient/client's blood pressure is 150/90 mmHg, which is above the expected limit and consistent with Stage I hypertension. Will monitor change in blood pressure at next encounter.
Reassessment after nutrition intervention	Significant progress toward expected limit. Patient/client's blood pressure is 135/82 mmHg.

Updated: 2011 Edition

Personal Data (CH-1.1)

Definition

General patient/client information such as age, gender, race/ethnicity, occupation, tobacco use, and physical disability

Nutrition Assessment:

Indicators

Age***
- Age in days (neonates)***
- Age in months (up to 36 months)***
- Age in years***
- Other (e.g., age adjusted)***

Gender***
- Female***
- Male***

Race/ethnicity***
- White***
- Black/African American***
- Hispanic ethnicity***
- Asian***
- Other (specify)***

Language***
- English***
- Spanish***
- Other (specify)***

Literacy factors***
- Language barrier***
- Low literacy***

Education***
- Years of education (Year of education)***

Role in family***
- Specify***(patient/client's reported role, e.g., mother, cousin, in the description of his/her family)

Tobacco use***
- Yes***
  - Average number cigarettes smoked per day (number/day)***
  - Total number of other tobacco products used/day (number/day)***
  - Number years tobacco products used on a regular basis (years)***
- No***

Physical disability***
- Eyesight impaired***
- Hearing impaired***
- Other (specify)***

Mobility***
- House bound***
- Bed or chair bound***
- Tremors (Parkinson's)***
- Other (specify)***

Examples of the measurement methods or data sources for these outcome indicators: Patient/client report, medical record, referring health care provider or agency, surveys, administrative data sets

Typically used with following domains of nutrition interventions: Food and/or Nutrient Delivery, nutrition education, nutrition counseling, coordination of nutrition care

*** Denotes indicator is used for nutrition assessment only. Other indicators are used for both nutrition assessment and nutrition monitoring and evaluation.*

Personal Data (CH-1.1)

Typically used to determine the following nutrition diagnoses: N/A

Clinical judgment must be used to select indicators and determine the appropriate measurement techniques and reference standards for a given patient population and setting. Once identified, these indicators, measurement techniques, and reference standards should be identified in policies and procedures or other documents for use in patient/client records, quality or performance improvement, or in formal research projects.

Evaluation

Criteria for Evaluation
Comparison to Goal or Reference Standard:
1) Goal (tailored to patient/client's needs)
   OR
2) Reference Standard

Patient/Client Example(s)
Example(s) of one or two of the Nutrition Care Indicators (includes sample initial assessment documentation for one of the indicators)

Indicator(s) Selected
Age, race/ethnicity, gender and education level

Criteria for Evaluation
Comparison to Goal or Reference Standard:
1) Goal: Not typically used
   OR
2) Reference Standard: No standard exists

Sample nutrition assessment documentation

Initial nutrition assessment with patient/client	Patient/client is a 40-year-old African American male with new onset type 2 diabetes, 7th grade education level

Patient/Client or Family Nutrition-Oriented Medical/Health History (CH-2.1)

Definition

Patient/client or family member disease states, conditions, and illnesses that may impact nutritional status

Nutrition Assessment

Indicators

Patient/client chief nutrition complaint (specify)***

Cardiovascular***
- Cardiovascular disease***
- Congestive heart failure***
- Hyperlipidemia***
- Hypertension***
- Stroke***
- Other***

Endocrine/metabolism***
- Cystic fibrosis***
- Diabetes mellitus***
- Diabetes, gestational***
- Inborn errors***
- Malnutrition/failure to thrive***
- Metabolic syndrome***
- Obesity***
- Overweight (specify duration)***
- Other (specify)***

Excretory***
- Dehydration***
- Renal failure, acute***
- Renal failure, chronic***
- Other (specify)***

Gastrointestinal***
- Crohn's disease***
- Diverticulitis/osis***
- Dyspepsia***
- Inflammatory bowel disease***
- Lactase deficiency***
- Liver disease***
- Pancreatic disease (specify)***
- Other (specify)***

Gynecological***
- Amenorrhea***
- Lactating***
- Mastitis***
- Perimenopausal/postmenopausal***
- Pregnant***
  - Gestational age (weeks)***
  - Single fetuses***
  - Multiple fetus (specify)***
- Other (specify)***

Hematology/oncology***
- Anemia (specify)***
- Cancer (specify)***
- Other (specify)***

Immune***
- AIDS/HIV***
- Food allergies***
- Sepsis/severe infection***
- Other (specify)***

Integumentary***
- Burns***
- Other (specify)***

Musculoskeletal***
- Multiple trauma/fractures***
- Osteoporosis***
- Other (specify)***

Neurological***
- Developmental delay***
- Other (specify) ***

Psychological***
- Alcoholism***
- Cognitive impairment***

*** Denotes indicator is used for nutrition assessment only. Other indicators are used for both nutrition assessment and nutrition monitoring and evaluation.*

4th Edition

ASSESSMENT/MON & EVAL

Patient/Client or Family Nutrition-Oriented Medical/Health History (CH-2.1)

- Dementia/Alzheimer's***
- Depression***
- Eating disorder (specify)***
- Psychosis***
- Other (specify)***

Respiratory***
- Chronic obstructive pulmonary disease***
- Other (specify)***

Other***

Examples of the measurement methods or data sources for these outcome indicators: Medical record, referring health care provider or agency

Typically used with following domains of nutrition interventions: Nutrition education, nutrition counseling

Typically used to determine the following nutrition diagnoses: All

Clinical judgment must be used to select indicators and determine the appropriate measurement techniques and reference standards for a given patient population and setting. Once identified, these indicators, measurement techniques, and reference standards should be identified in policies and procedures or other documents for use in patient/client records, quality or performance improvement, or in formal research projects.

Evaluation

Criteria for Evaluation
Comparison to Goal or Reference Standard:
1) Goal (tailored to patient/client's needs)
   OR
2) Reference Standard

Patient Example(s)
Example(s) of one or two of the Nutrition Care Indicators (includes sample initial assessment documentation for one of the indicators)

Indicator(s) Selected
Cardiovascular disease (CVD)

Criteria for Evaluation
Comparison to Goal or Reference Standard:
1) Goal: Not typically used
   OR
2) Reference Standard: No reference standard exists.

Sample nutrition assessment documentation

Initial nutrition assessment with patient/client	Patient/client with history of CVD. Recommend the Therapeutic Lifestyle Changes (TLC) diet in accordance with the reference standard (e.g., NHLBI Adult Treatment Panel III guidelines)

Updated: 2011 Edition

*** Denotes indicator is used for nutrition assessment only. Other indicators are used for both nutrition assessment and nutrition monitoring and evaluation.*

Treatments/Therapy (CH-2.2)

Definition

Documented medical or surgical treatments that may impact nutritional status of the patient

Nutrition Assessment

Indicators

Medical treatment/therapy***

- Chemotherapy***
- Dialysis***
- Mechanical ventilation/oxygen therapy***
- Ostomy (specify)***
- Radiation therapy***
- Other (specify, e.g., speech, OT, PT)***

Surgical treatment***

- Coronary artery bypass (CABG)***
- Gastric bypass (specify type)***
- Intestinal resection***
- Joint/orthopedic surgery/replacement***
- Limb amputation***
- Organ transplant (specify)***
- Total gastrectomy***
- Other (specify)***

Palliative/end-of-life care (care of patient/client with terminal or life-threatening conditions)***

Examples of the measurement methods or data sources for these indicators: Patient/client interview, medical record, referring health care provider or agency

Typically used with following domains of nutrition interventions: Food and/or nutrient delivery, nutrition education, nutrition counseling, coordination of nutrition care

Typically used to determine the following nutrition diagnoses: Impaired nutrient utilization, increased nutrient needs, altered gastrointestinal function, biting/chewing (masticatory) difficulty, involuntary weight loss.

Clinical judgment must be used to select indicators and determine the appropriate measurement techniques and reference standards for a given patient population and setting. Once identified, these indicators, measurement techniques, and reference standards should be identified in policies and procedures or other documents for use in patient/client records, quality or performance improvement, or in formal research projects.

*** Denotes indicator is used for nutrition assessment only. Other indicators are used for both nutrition assessment and nutrition monitoring and evaluation.*

ASSESSMENT/MON & EVAL

Treatments/Therapy (CH-2.2)

Evaluation

Criteria for Evaluation

Comparison to Goal or Reference Standard:
1) Goal (tailored to patient/client's needs)
   OR
2) Reference Standard

Patient/Client Example(s)

Example(s) of one or two of the Nutrition Care Indicators (includes sample initial assessment documentation for one of the indicators)

Indicator(s) Selected

Radiation therapy

Criteria for Evaluation

Comparison to Goal or Reference Standard:
1) Goal: Patient/client receiving radiation therapy for lung cancer, experiencing decreased appetite and pain with eating. Goal is to optimize nutrition during radiation therapy.
   OR
2) Reference Standard: No standards exist.

Sample nutrition assessment documentation

Initial nutrition assessment with patient/client	Patient/client receiving radiation therapy for lung cancer, experiencing decreased appetite due to fatigue and pain with eating.

Social History (CH-3.1)

Definition

Patient/client information such as socioeconomic factors, housing situation, medical support, occupation, religion, history of recent crisis and involvement in social groups

Nutrition Assessment

Indicators

Socioeconomic factors***
- Economic constraints (major/minor)***
- Access to medical care (full/limited/none)***
- Diverts food money to other needs***
- Other (specify)***

Living/housing situation***
- Lives alone***
- Lives with family member/caregiver***
- Homeless***

Domestic issues***
- Specify***

Social and medical support***
- Family members***
- Caregivers***
- Community group/senior center/church***
- Support group attendance (e.g., weight control, substance abuse, etc.)***
- Other (specify)***

Geographic location of home***
- Urban***
- Rural***

- Limited exposure to sunlight (vitamin D)***
- Other (specify)***

Occupation***
- Stay-at-home mother***
- Student***
- Retired***
- Specify***

Religion***
- Catholic***
- Jewish***
- Protestant***
  Specify***
- Islam***
- Specify***

History of recent crisis***
- Job loss***
- Family member death***
- Trauma, surgery***
- Other (specify)***

Daily stress level (high, moderate, low bodily or mental tension)***

Examples of the measurement methods or data sources for these outcome indicators: Patient/client report, medical record, referring health care provider or agency

Typically used with following domains of nutrition interventions: Food and/or nutrient delivery, nutrition education, nutrition counseling, coordination of nutrition care

*** *Denotes indicator is used for nutrition assessment only. Other indicators are used for both nutrition assessment and nutrition monitoring and evaluation.*

Social History (CH-3.1)

Typically used to determine the following nutrition diagnoses: All

Clinical judgment must be used to select indicators and determine the appropriate measurement techniques and reference standards for a given patient population and setting. Once identified, these indicators, measurement techniques, and reference standards should be identified in policies and procedures or other documents for use in patient/client records, quality or performance improvement, or in formal research projects.

Evaluation

Criteria for Evaluation

Comparison to Goal or Reference Standard:
1) Goal (tailored to patient/client's needs)
   OR
2) Reference Standard

Patient/Client Example(s)

Example(s) of one or two of the Nutrition Care Indicators (includes sample initial assessment documentation for one of the indicators)

Indicator(s) Selected

Age, race/ethnicity, and gender

Criteria for Evaluation

Comparison to Goal or Reference Standard:
1) Goal: Not typically used
   OR
2) Reference Standard: No reference standard exists.

Sample nutrition assessment documentation

Initial nutrition assessment with patient/client	Patient/client is house bound, lives in a rural area, and receives one meal/day from Meals on Wheels.

Estimated Energy Needs (CS-1.1)

Definition

Estimated quantity of total energy needed for nutritional adequacy.

Purpose

Identify appropriate reference standard of energy intake needs for individual patients/clients. Utilized as a basis of comparison to assess adequacy or excessiveness of patient/client's estimated total energy intake as compared to estimated needs and for development of the nutrition prescription.

Indicators

Total estimated energy needs assumed to be consistent with the Dietary Reference Intakes unless otherwise specified: (specify, e.g., calories/day, calories/kg/day)

	EAR	RDA	AI	UL	Other
Energy*					Formula

EAR — Estimated Average Requirement
RDA — Recommended Dietary Allowance
AI   — Adequate Intake
UL   — Tolerable Upper Intake Level

*See DRI interpretation table (page 84) of the International Dietetics and Nutrition Terminology (IDNT)Reference Manual, Fourth Edition.

Method for estimating energy needs:

- Estimated (specify, e.g., patient/client goal or nutrition prescription, equation/method and adjustments for activity, stress, pregnancy, breastfeeding, and/or fever)
- Measured (specify assessment method)

  Note: Comparison to the Dietary Reference Intakes is assumed, but other reference intake
  standards may be used.

Estimated Fat Needs (CS-2.1)

Definition
Estimated quantity of total and/or type fat intake needed for nutritional adequacy.

Purpose
Identify appropriate reference standard of fat intake needs for individual patients/clients. Utilized as a basis of comparison to assess adequacy or excessiveness of patient/client's estimated total fat intake as compared to needs and for development of the nutrition prescription.

Indicators

Total fat needs, assumed to be consistent with the Dietary Reference Intakes unless otherwise specified: (specify, e.g., grams/day, grams/kg/day, percent of calories)

Types of fat needed (specify, e.g., grams/day, grams/kg/day, percent of calories)

Macronutrients*	EAR	RDA	AI	UL	Other
Fat			X Infants only		Acceptable Macronutrient Distribution Range (AMDR) (children and adults)
n-6 polyunsaturated fatty acids (linoleic acid)			X (All ages)		Acceptable Macronutrient Distribution Range (AMDR) (children and adults)
n-3 polyunsaturated fatty acids (α-linolenic acid)			X (All ages)		
Dietary cholesterol Trans fatty acids Saturated fatty acids					As low as possible while consuming a nutritionally adequate diet

EAR — Estimated Average Requirement
RDA — Recommended Dietary Allowance
AI — Adequate Intake
UL — Tolerable Upper Intake Level

*See DRI interpretation table (page 84) of the International Dietetics and Nutrition Terminology (IDNT)Reference Manual, Fourth Edition.

Method for estimating fat needs (specify, e.g., patient/client goal or nutrition prescription, disease/condition-based reference standard, Dietary Reference Intake)

Note: Comparison to the Dietary Reference Intakes is assumed, but other reference intake standards may be used.

Estimated Protein Needs (CS-2.2)

Definition

Estimated quantity and/or type of protein needed for nutritional adequacy.

Purpose

Identify appropriate reference standard of protein intake needs for individual patients/clients. Utilized as a basis of comparison to assess adequacy or excessiveness of patient/client's estimated total protein intake as compared to estimated needs and for development of the nutrition prescription.

Indicators

Total estimated protein needs, assumed to be consistent with the Dietary Reference Intakes unless otherwise specified: (specify, e.g., grams/day, grams/kg/day, percent of calories)

Macronutrient*	EAR	RDA	AI	UL	Other
Protein	X All except infants 0 to 6 months	X All except infants 0 to 6 months	X Infants 0 to 6 months		Acceptable Macronutrient Distribution Range (children and adults)

EAR — Estimated Average Requirement
RDA — Recommended Dietary Allowance
AI — Adequate Intake
UL — Tolerable Upper Intake Level

*See DRI interpretation table (page 84) of the International Dietetics and Nutrition Terminology (IDNT)Reference Manual, Fourth Edition.

Types of protein/amino acids needed (specify, e.g., grams/day, grams/kg/day, percent of total protein, percent of calories)

Method for estimating protein needs (specify, e.g., patient/client goal or nutrition prescription, disease/condition-based reference standard, Dietary Reference Intake)

Note: Comparison to the Dietary Reference Intakes is assumed, but other reference intake standards may be used.

Estimated Carbohydrate Needs (CS-2.3)

Definition
Estimated quantity of total and/or type of carbohydrates needed for nutritional adequacy.

Purpose
Identify appropriate reference standard of carbohydrate intake needs for individual patients/clients. Utilized for assessing the adequacy or excessiveness of patient/client's estimated total carbohydrate intake as compared to estimated needs and for development of the nutrition prescription.

Indicators
Total estimated carbohydrate needs assumed to be consistent with the Dietary Reference Intakes unless otherwise specified: (specify, e.g., grams/day, grams or mg/kg/min, percent of calories)

Types of carbohydrate needed (specify, e.g., grams/day, grams or mg/kg/min, percent of carbohydrate, percent of calories)

Macronutrients*	EAR	RDA	AI	UL	Other
Carbohydrates		X	X infants		Acceptable Macronutrient Distribution Range (children and adults)
					Added sugars – limit to no more than 25% of total energy (all ages)

EAR — Estimated Average Requirement
RDA — Recommended Dietary Allowance
AI — Adequate Intake
UL — Tolerable Upper Intake Level

See DRI interpretation table (page 84) of the International Dietetics and Nutrition Terminology (IDNT)Reference Manual, Fourth Edition.

Method for estimating carbohydrate needs (specify, e.g., patient/client goal or nutrition prescription, disease/condition-based reference standard, Dietary Reference Intake)

Note: Comparison to the Dietary Reference Intakes is assumed, but other reference intake standards may be used.

Estimated Fiber Needs (CS-2.4)

Definition

Estimated quantity of total and/or type of fiber needed for nutritional adequacy.

Purpose

Identify appropriate reference standard of fiber intake needs for individual patients/clients. Utilized as a basis of comparison to assess adequacy or excessiveness of patient/client's estimated total fiber intake as compared to estimated needs and for development of the nutrition prescription.

Indicators

Total estimated fiber needs, assumed to be consistent with the Dietary Reference Intakes unless otherwise specified: (specify, e.g., grams/day, grams/1000 kcal/day)

Macronutrients*	EAR	RDA	AI	UL	Other
Fiber			X Children and adults		

EAR — Estimated Average Requirement
RDA — Recommended Dietary Allowance
AI — Adequate Intake
UL — Tolerable Upper Intake Level

*See DRI interpretation table (page 84) of the International Dietetics and Nutrition Terminology (IDNT)Reference Manual, Fourth Edition.

Types of fiber needed (specify, e.g., grams/day, percent of total fiber)

Method for estimating fiber needs (specify, e.g., patient/client goal or nutrition prescription, disease/condition-based reference standard, Dietary Reference Intake)

Note: Comparison to the Dietary Reference Intakes is assumed, but other reference intake standards may be used.

Estimated Fluid Needs (CS-3.1)

Definition
Estimated quantity of fluid needed for nutritional adequacy.

Purpose
Identify appropriate reference standard of fluid intake needs for individual patients/clients. Utilized as a basis of comparison to assess adequacy or excessiveness of patient/client's estimated total fluid intake as compared to estimated need and for development of the nutrition prescription.

Indicators

Total estimated fluid needs, assumed to be consistent with the Dietary Reference Intakes unless otherwise specified: (specify, e.g., mL or L/day, mL/kg/day, mL/calories expended, mL/m^2/day, mL output)

Macronutrient*	EAR	RDA	AI	UL	Other
Total Water			X		

EAR — Estimated Average Requirement
RDA — Recommended Dietary Allowance
AI — Adequate Intake
UL — Tolerable Upper Intake Level

*See DRI interpretation table (page 84) of the International Dietetics and Nutrition Terminology (IDNT)Reference Manual, Fourth Edition.

Method for estimating fluid needs (specify, e.g., patient/client goal or nutrition prescription, disease/condition-based reference standard, Dietary Reference Intake and adjustments, if needed, e.g., patient/client goal or nutrition prescription, increased due to fever, sweating, hyperventilation, hyperthyroid, extraordinary gastric/renal losses, or decreased due to, for example, renal or liver disease)

Note:Comparison to the Dietary Reference Intakes is assumed, but other reference intake standards may be used.

Estimated Vitamin Needs (CS-4.1)

Definition
Estimated quantity of one or more vitamins needed for nutritional adequacy and avoidance of toxicity.

Purpose
Identify appropriate reference standard of vitamin intake needs for individual patients/clients. Utilized as a basis of comparison to assess adequacy or excessiveness of patient/client's estimated total vitamin intake as compared to estimated needs and for development of the nutrition prescription.

Indicators
Total estimated vitamin needs, assumed to be consistent with the Dietary Reference Intakes unless otherwise specified:

Micronutrients— Vitamins*	EAR	RDA	AI	UL
Vitamin A (µg/day)	X	X	X Infants	X
Vitamin C (mg/day)	X	X	X Infants	X Children and adults
Vitamin D (µg/day)			X	X
Vitamin E (mg/day)	X	X	X Infants	X Children and adults
Vitamin K (µg/day)			X	
Thiamin (mg/day)	X	X	X Infants	
Riboflavin (mg/day)	X	X	X Infants	
Niacin (mg/day)	X	X	X Infants	X Children and adults
Vitamin B6 (mg/day)	X	X	X Infants	X Children and adults
Folate (µg/day)	X	X	X Infants	X Children and adults
Vitamin B12 (µg/day)	X	X	X Infants	

Estimated Vitamin Needs (CS-4.1)

Indicators, cont'd

Micronutrients—Vitamins*, cont'd	EAR	RDA	AI	UL
Pantothenic acid (mg/day)			X	
Biotin (µg/day)			X	
Choline (mg/d)			X	X Children and adults

EAR — Estimated Average Requirement
RDA — Recommended Dietary Allowance
AI — Adequate Intake
UL — Tolerable Upper Intake Level

See DRI interpretation table (page 84) of the International Dietetics and Nutrition Terminology (IDNT)Reference Manual, Fourth Edition.

Method for estimating vitamin needs (specify, e.g., patient/client goal or nutrition prescription, disease/condition-based reference standard, any adjustments for special conditions or situations, Dietary Reference Intake)

Note:Comparison to the Dietary Reference Intakes is assumed, but other reference intake standards may be used.

Estimated Mineral/Element Needs (CS-4.2)

Definition

Estimated quantity of one or more minerals needed for nutritional adequacy and avoidance of toxicity.

Purpose

Identify appropriate reference standard of mineral intake needs for individual patients/clients. Utilized as a basis of comparison to assess adequacy or excessiveness of patient/client's estimated mineral intake as compared to estimated needs and for development of the nutrition prescription.

Indicators

Total estimated mineral needs, assumed to be consistent with the Dietary Reference Intakes unless otherwise specified:

Micronutrients—Minerals/elements*	EAR	RDA	AI	UL	Other
Calcium (mg/day)			X	X Children and adults	
Chloride (g/day)			X	X Children and adults	
Chromium (µg/day)			X		
Copper (µg/day)	X	X	X Infants	X Children and adults	
Fluoride (mg/day)			X	X	
Iodine (µg/day)	X	X	X Infants	X Children and adults	
Iron (mg/day)	X	X	X Infants 0-6 mos.	X	
Magnesium (mg/day)	X	X	X Infants	X Children and adults	

Estimated Mineral/Element Needs (CS-4.2)

Indicators, cont'd

Micronutrients— Minerals/ elements,* cont'd	EAR	RDA	AI	UL	Other
Manganese (mg/d)			X	X Children and adults	
Molybdenum (mg/day)	X Children and adults	X Children and adults	X Infants	X Children and adults	
Phosphorus (mg/ day)	X	X	X Infants	X Children and adults	
Potassium (g/day)			X		
Selenium (μg/day)	X	X	X Infants	X	
Sodium (g/day)			X	X Children and adults	
Sulfate (g/day)	X	X	X Infants	X	
Zinc (mg/day)	X	X	X Infants 0 to 6 mos.	X	

EAR — Estimated Average Requirement
RDA — Recommended Dietary Allowance
AI — Adequate Intake
UL — Tolerable Upper Intake Level

*See DRI interpretation table (page 84) of the International Dietetics and Nutrition Terminology (IDNT)Reference Manual, Fourth Edition.

Method for estimating mineral needs (specify, e.g., patient/client goal or nutrition prescription, disease/condition-based reference standard, any adjustments for special conditions or situations, Dietary Reference Intake)

Note:Comparison to the Dietary Reference Intakes is assumed, but other reference intake standards may be used.

Recommended Body Weight/Body Mass Index/Growth (5.1)

Definition

Estimated reference ideal body weight (known as desirable body weight), body mass index, and/or growth parameter used to evaluate nutritional status

Purpose

Identify appropriate reference standard for body weight for individual patients/clients. Utilized as a basis of comparison to assess patient/client's body weight as compared to recommendations and for development of the nutrition prescription

Indicators (Measures)

Ideal/reference body weight†

- Method for determining ideal body weight (IBW)/desirable body weight (specify, e.g., Hamwi equation, growth chart)
- IBW adjustment (e.g., spinal cord injury, amputees)
- % IBW
- Adjusted body weight/metabolically active weight for overweight/obesity (specify, e.g., equation)

Recommended Body Mass Index (BMI)* (kg/m2)

- Normal range BMI (specify if using, e.g., adjustment for South East Asian body types)

Desired growth pattern (based on individual health, growth pattern, and genetic potential)

- 0 to 36 months
  - Weight-for-age (percentile rank)
  - Length-for-age (percentile rank)
  - Weight-for-length (percentile rank)
  - Head circumference-for-age (percentile rank)
- 2 to 5 years
  - Weight-for-stature (percentile rank)
- 2 to 20 years
  - Weight-for-age (percentile rank)
  - Stature-for-age (percentile rank)
  - BMI-for-age (percentile rank)
- Specialized and disease-specific growth charts (specify, e.g., type chart and percentile rank)

  Note: Estimated stature and corrected age for prematurity are found on the Body Composition/Growth/Weight History reference sheet.

  †Please refer to the Academy Evidence Analysis Library, Energy Expenditure: Measurement vs. Estimation Evidence Analysis Project (2006), available at: http://www.andevidence library.com/topic.cfm?cat=1151, for recommendations related to using actual weight versus IBW or ABW for estimating energy expenditure.

  *BMI is a measure of the weight of an individual scaled according to height. It is a common method for assessing body fat in the clinical setting and is compared to a population reference standard (e.g., US National Institutes of Health guidelines or World Health Organization guidelines). BMI was designed for use within a physically inactive population.

Updated: 2011 Edition

NCP Step 2: Nutrition Diagnosis

What is the purpose of a nutrition diagnosis? The purpose is to identify and describe a specific nutrition problem that can be resolved or improved through treatment/ nutrition intervention by a food and nutrition professional. A nutrition diagnosis (e.g., inconsistent carbohydrate intake) is different from a medical diagnosis (e.g., diabetes).

How does a food and nutrition professional determine a nutrition diagnosis? Food and nutrition professionals use the data collected in the nutrition assessment to identify and label the patient/client's* nutrition diagnosis using standard nutrition diagnostic terminology. Each nutrition diagnosis has a reference sheet that includes its definition, possible etiology/causes, and common signs or symptoms identified in the nutrition assessment step.

How are the nutrition diagnoses organized? In three categories:

> **Intake**—*Too much or too little of a food or nutrient compared to actual or estimated needs*
>
> **Clinical**—*Nutrition problems that relate to medical or physical conditions*
>
> **Behavioral-Environmental**—*Knowledge, attitudes, beliefs, physical environment, access to food, or food safety*

How is the nutrition diagnosis documented? Food and nutrition professionals write a PES statement to describe the problem, its root cause, and the assessment data that provide evidence for the nutrition diagnosis. The format for the PES statement is "Nutrition problem label related to _____ as evidenced by _____."

> **(P) Problem or Nutrition Diagnosis Label**—Describes alterations in the patient/client's nutritional status.
>
> **(E) Etiology**—Cause/Contributing Risk Factors (Linked to the nutrition diagnosis label by the words "related to.")
>
> **(S) Signs/Symptoms**—Data used to determine that the patient/client has the nutrition diagnosis specified. (Linked to the etiology by the words "as evidenced by.")

No nutrition diagnosis at this time (NO-1.1) may be documented if the assessment indicates that no nutrition problem currently exists that warrants a nutrition intervention.

What are the guidelines for selecting the nutrition diagnosis and writing a clear PES statement? The most important and urgent problem to be addressed is selected. When specifying the nutrition diagnosis and writing the PES statement, food and nutrition professionals ask themselves a series of questions that help clarify the nutrition diagnosis. (See the critical thinking box.)

DIAGNOSIS

Patient/client refers to individuals, groups, populations, family members, and/or caregivers.

4th Edition

Critical thinking during this step...

Evaluate your PES statement by using the following:

P – Can the nutrition professional resolve or improve the nutrition diagnosis for this individual, group, or population? When all things are equal and there is a choice between stating the PES statement using two nutrition diagnoses from different domains, consider the Intake nutrition diagnosis as the one more specific to the role of the RD.

E – Evaluate what you have used as your etiology to determine if it is the "root cause" or the most specific root cause that the RD can address with a nutrition intervention. If as an RD you cannot resolve the problem by addressing the etiology, can the RD intervention at least lessen the signs and symptoms?

S – Will measuring the signs and symptoms indicate if the problem is resolved or improved? Are the signs and symptoms specific enough that you can monitor (measure/evaluate changes) and document resolution or improvement of the nutrition diagnosis?

PES Overall – Does the nutrition assessment data support a particular nutrition diagnosis with a typical etiology and signs and symptoms?

Are food and nutrition professionals limited to the nutrition diagnosis terms?
Nutrition diagnosis terms and definitions were developed with extensive input and should fit most situations; however, food and nutrition professionals can submit proposals for additions or revisions using the Procedure for Nutrition Controlled Vocabulary/Terminology Maintenance/Review available from the Academy.

Detailed information about this step can be found in the Academy of Nutrition and Dietetics' International Dietetics and Nutrition Terminology (IDNT) Reference Manual: Standardized Language for the Nutrition Care Process, Fourth Edition.

4th Edition   148

Nutrition Diagnostic Terminology

Each term has an Academy unique identifier, a five-digit number (e.g., 99999) following the alpha-numeric IDNT code. Neither should be visible in nutrition documentation. The Academy unique identifier is for data tracking purposes in electronic records.

INTAKE NI

Defined as "actual problems related to intake of energy, nutrients, fluids, bioactive substances through oral diet or nutrition support"

Energy Balance (1)

Defined as "actual or estimated changes in energy (calorie/kcal/kJ) balance"

- ❑ Increased energy expenditure — NI-1.1 — 10633
- ❑ Inadequate energy intake — NI-1.2 — 10634
- ❑ Excessive energy intake — NI-1.3 — 10635
- ❑ Predicted suboptimal energy intake — NI-1.4 — 10636
- ❑ Predicted excessive energy intake — NI-1.5 — 10637

Oral or Nutrition Support Intake (2)

Defined as "actual or estimated food and beverage intake from oral diet or nutrition support compared with patient goal"

- ❑ Inadequate oral intake — NI-2.1 — 10639
- ❑ Excessive oral intake — NI-2.2 — 10640
- ❑ Inadequate enteral nutrition infusion — NI-2.3 — 10641
- ❑ Excessive enteral nutrition infusion — NI-2.4 — 10642
- ❑ Less than optimal enteral nutrition composition or modality — NI-2.5 — 10852
- ❑ Inadequate parenteral nutrition infusion — NI-2.6 — 10644
- ❑ Excessive parenteral nutrition infusion — NI-2.7 — 10645
- ❑ Less than optimal parenteral nutrition composition or modality — NI-2.8 — 10853
- ❑ Limited food acceptance — NI-2.9 — 10647

Fluid Intake (3)

Defined as "actual or estimated fluid intake compared with patient goal"

- ❑ Inadequate fluid intake — NI-3.1 — 10649
- ❑ Excessive fluid intake — NI-3.2 — 10650

Bioactive Substances (4)

Defined as "actual or observed intake of bioactive substances, including single or multiple functional food components, ingredients, dietary supplements, alcohol"

- ❑ Inadequate bioactive substance intake (*specify*)_____ — NI-4.1 — 10652
- ❑ Excessive bioactive substance intake (*specify*)_____ — NI-4.2 — 10653
- ❑ Excessive alcohol intake — NI-4.3 — 10654

Nutrient (5)

Defined as "actual or estimated intake of specific nutrient groups or single nutrients as compared with desired levels"

- ❑ Increased nutrient needs (*specify*) _____ — NI-5.1 — 10656
- ❑ Malnutrition — NI-5.2 — 10657
- ❑ Inadequate protein-energy intake — NI-5.3 — 10658
- ❑ Decreased nutrient needs (*specify*) _____ — NI-5.4 — 10659
- ❑ Imbalance of nutrients — NI-5.5 — 10660

Fat and Cholesterol (5.6)

- ❑ Inadequate fat intake — NI-5.6.1 — 10662
- ❑ Excessive fat intake — NI-5.6.2 — 10663
- ❑ Less than optimal intake of types of fats (*specify*)_____ — NI-5.6.3 — 10854

Protein (5.7)

- ❑ Inadequate protein intake — NI-5.7.1 — 10666
- ❑ Excessive protein intake — NI-5.7.2 — 10667
- ❑ Less than optimal intake of types of proteins or amino acids (*specify*) _____ — NI-5.7.3 — 10855

Carbohydrate and Fiber (5.8)

- ❑ Inadequate carbohydrate intake — NI-5.8.1 — 10670
- ❑ Excessive carbohydrate intake — NI-5.8.2 — 10671
- ❑ Less than optimal intake of types of carbohydrate (*specify*) _____ — NI-5.8.3 — 10856
- ❑ Inconsistent carbohydrate intake — NI-5.8.4 — 10673
- ❑ Inadequate fiber intake — NI-5.8.5 — 10675
- ❑ Excessive fiber intake — NI-5.8.6 — 10676

Vitamin (5.9)

- ❑ Inadequate vitamin intake (*specify*) — NI-5.9.1
  - ❑ A (1) — 10679
  - ❑ C (2) — 10680
  - ❑ D (3) — 10681
  - ❑ E (4) — 10682
  - ❑ K (5) — 10683
  - ❑ Thiamin (6) — 10684
  - ❑ Riboflavin (7) — 10685
  - ❑ Niacin (8) — 10686
  - ❑ Folate (9) — 10687
  - ❑ B6 (10) — 10688
  - ❑ B12 (11) — 10689
  - ❑ Pantothenic acid (12) — 10690
  - ❑ Biotin (13) — 10691

□ Excessive vitamin intake   NI-5.9.2
(*specify*)

□ A (1)		10694
□ C (2)		10695
□ D (3)		10696
□ E (4)		10697
□ K (5)		10698
□ Thiamin (6)		10699
□ Riboflavin (7)		10700
□ Niacin (8)		10701
□ Folate (9)		10702
□ B6 (10)		10703
□ B12 (11)		10704
□ Pantothenic acid (12)		10705
□ Biotin (13)		10706

Mineral (5.10)

□ Inadequate mineral intake NI-5.10.1
(*specify*)

□ Calcium (1)	10710
□ Chloride (2)	10711
□ Iron (3)	10712
□ Magnesium (4)	10713
□ Potassium (5)	10714
□ Phosphorus (6)	10715
□ Sodium (7)	10716
□ Zinc (8)	10717
□ Sulfate (9)	10718
□ Fluoride (10)	10719
□ Copper (11)	10720
□ Iodine (12)	10721
□ Selenium (13)	10722
□ Manganese (14)	10723
□ Chromium (15)	10724
□ Molybdenum (16)	10725
□ Boron (17)	10726
□ Cobalt (18)	10727

□ Excessive mineral intake NI-5.10.2
(*specify*)

□ Calcium (1)	10730
□ Chloride (2)	10731
□ Iron (3)	10732
□ Magnesium (4)	10733
□ Potassium (5)	10734
□ Phosphorus (6)	10735
□ Sodium (7)	10736
□ Zinc (8)	10737
□ Sulfate (9)	10738
□ Fluoride (10)	10739
□ Copper (11)	10740
□ Iodine (12)	10741
□ Selenium (13)	10742
□ Manganese (14)	10743
□ Chromium (15)	10744
□ Molybdenum (16)	10745
□ Boron (17)	10746
□ Cobalt (18)	10747

Multi-nutrient (5.11)

□ Predicted suboptimal	NI-5.11.1	10750
nutrient intake (*specify*) _____		

□ Predicted excessive	NI-5.11.2	10751
nutrient intake (*specify*) _____		

CLINICAL   NC
Defined as "nutritional findings/problems identified that relate to medical or physical conditions"

Functional (1)
Defined as "change in physical or mechanical functioning that interferes with or prevents desired nutritional consequences"

□ Swallowing difficulty	NC-1.1	10754
□ Biting/Chewing (masticatory) difficulty	NC-1.2	10755
□ Breastfeeding difficulty	NC-1.3	10756
□ Altered GI function	NC-1.4	10757

Biochemical (2)
Defined as "change in capacity to metabolize nutrients as a result of medications, surgery, or as indicated by altered lab values"

□ Impaired nutrient utilization	NC-2.1	10759
□ Altered nutrition-related laboratory values (*specify*) _____	NC-2.2	10760
□ Food–medication interaction (*specify*) _____	NC-2.3	10761
□ Predicted food– medication interaction (*specify*)____	NC-2.4	10762

Weight (3)
Defined as "chronic weight or changed weight status when compared with usual or desired body weight"

□ Underweight	NC-3.1	10764
□ Unintended weight loss	NC-3.2	10765
□ Overweight/obesity	NC-3.3	
□ Overweight, adult or pediatric (1)		10767
□ Obese, pediatric (2)		10768
□ Obese, Class I (3)		10769
□ Obese, Class II (4)		10818
□ Obese, Class III (5)		10819
□ Unintended weight gain	NC-3.4	10770
□ Suboptimal growth rate	NC-3.5	10802
□ Excessive growth rate	NC-3.6	10803

BEHAVIORAL-ENVIRONMENTAL NB
Defined as "nutritional findings/problems identified that relate to knowledge, attitudes/beliefs, physical environment, access to food, or food safety"

Knowledge and Beliefs (1)
Defined as "actual knowledge and beliefs as related, observed, or documented"

□ Food- and nutrition-related knowledge deficit	NB-1.1	10773
□ Unsupported beliefs/ attitudes about food-or nutrition-related topics (use with caution)	NB-1.2	10857
□ Not ready for diet/lifestyle change	NB-1.3	10775
□ Self-monitoring deficit	NB-1.4	10776

☐ Disordered eating pattern	NB-1.5	10777
☐ Limited adherence to nutrition-related recommendations	NB-1.6	10778
☐ Undesirable food choices	NB-1.7	10779

Physical Activity and Function (2)

Defined as "actual physical activity, self-care, and quality-of-life problems as reported, observed, or documented"

☐ Physical inactivity	NB-2.1	10782
☐ Excessive physical activity	NB-2.2	10783
☐ Inability to manage self-care	NB-2.3	10780
☐ Impaired ability to prepare foods/meals	NB-2.4	10785
☐ Poor nutrition quality of life	NB-2.5	10786
☐ Self-feeding difficulty	NB-2.6	10787

Food Safety and Access (3)

Defined as "actual problems with food safety or access to food, water, or nutrition-related supplies"

☐ Intake of unsafe food	NB-3.1	10789
☐ Limited access to food or water	NB-3.2	10790
☐ Limited access to nutrition-related supplies	NB-3.3	10791

OTHER   NO

Defined as "nutrition findings that are not classified as intake, clinical or behavioral-environmental problems."

Other (1)

| ☐ No nutrition diagnosis at this time | NO-1.1 | 10795 |

DIAGNOSIS

Increased Energy Expenditure (NI-1.1)

Definition

Resting metabolic rate (RMR) more than predicted requirements due to body composition; medications; or endocrine, neurologic, or genetic changes.

> *Note:RMR is the sum of metabolic processes of active cell mass related to the maintenance of normal body functions and regulatory balance during rest.*

Etiology (Cause/Contributing Risk Factors)

Factors gathered during the nutrition assessment process that contribute to the existence or the maintenance of pathophysiological, psychosocial, situational, developmental, cultural, and/or environmental problems:

- Physiological causes increasing nutrient needs due to anabolism, growth, maintenance of body temperature
- Voluntary or involuntary physical activity/movement

Signs/Symptoms (Defining Characteristics)

A typical cluster of subjective and objective signs and symptoms gathered during the nutrition assessment process that provide evidence that a problem exists; quantify the problem and describe its severity.

Nutrition Assessment Category	Potential Indicators of This Nutrition Diagnosis (one or more must be present)
Biochemical Data, Medical Tests and Procedures	
Anthropometric Measurements	• Unintentional weight loss of ≥ 10% in 6 months, ≥ 5% in 1 month (adults and pediatrics), and > 2% in 1 week (pediatrics) • Evidence of need for accelerated or catch-up growth or weight gain in children; absence of normal growth • Increased proportion of lean body mass
Nutrition-Focused Physical Findings	• Fever • Measured RMR > estimated or expected RMR
Food/Nutrition-Related History	• Increased physical activity, e.g., endurance athlete • Medications that increase energy expenditure
Client History	• Conditions associated with a diagnosis or treatment, e.g., Parkinson's disease, cerebral palsy, Alzheimer's disease, cystic fibrosis, chronic obstructive pulmonary disease (COPD)

DIAGNOSIS

Updated: 2013 Edition

4th Edition

Inadequate* Energy Intake (NI-1.2)

Definition
Energy intake that is less than energy expenditure, established reference standards, or recommendations based on physiological needs.

> *Note: May not be an appropriate nutrition diagnosis when the goal is weight loss, during end-of-life care, upon initiation of EN/PN, or acute stressed state (e.g., surgery, organ failure).*
>
> *Whenever possible, nutrient intake data should be considered in combination with clinical, biochemical, anthropometric information, medical diagnosis, clinical status, and/or other factors as well as diet to provide a valid assessment of nutritional status based on a totality of the evidence. (Institute of Medicine. Dietary Reference Intakes: Applications in Dietary Assessment. Washington, DC: National Academies Press; 2000.)*

Etiology (Cause/Contributing Risk Factors)
Factors gathered during the nutrition assessment process that contribute to the existence or the maintenance of pathophysiological, psychosocial, situational, developmental, cultural, and/or environmental problems:

- Pathological or physiological causes that result in increased energy requirements, e.g., increased nutrient needs due to prolonged catabolic illness
- Decreased ability to consume sufficient energy
- Lack of access to food or artificial nutrition, e.g., economic constraints, restricting food given to elderly and/or children
- Cultural practices that affect ability to access food
- Food- and nutrition-related knowledge deficit concerning energy intake
- Psychological causes such as depression and disordered eating

Signs/Symptoms (Defining Characteristics)
A typical cluster of subjective and objective signs and symptoms gathered during the nutrition assessment process that provide evidence that a problem exists; quantify the problem and describe its severity.

Nutrition Assessment Category	Potential Indicators of This Nutrition Diagnosis (one or more must be present)
Biochemical Data, Medical Tests and Procedures	
Anthropometric Measurements	• Failure to gain or maintain appropriate weight
Nutrition-Focused Physical Findings	• Poor dentition

*If a synonym for the term "inadequate" is helpful or needed, an approved alternate is the word "suboptimal."

Inadequate* Energy Intake (NI-1.2)

Food/Nutrition-Related History	Reports or observations of: • Estimated energy intake from diet less than needs based on estimated or measured resting metabolic rate • Restriction or omission of energy-dense foods from diet • Food avoidance and/or lack of interest in food • Inability to independently consume foods/fluids (diminished joint mobility of wrist, hand, or digits) • Estimated parenteral or enteral nutrition intake insufficient to meet needs based on estimated or measured resting metabolic rate • Excessive consumption of alcohol or other drugs that reduce hunger • Medications that affect appetite
Client History	• Conditions associated with diagnosis or treatment, e.g., mental illness, eating disorders, dementia, alcoholism, substance abuse, and acute or chronic pain management

Updated: 2013 Edition

*If a synonym for the term "inadequate" is helpful or needed, an approved alternate is the word "suboptimal."

4th Edition

Excessive Energy Intake (NI-1.3)

Definition
Energy intake that exceeds energy expenditure, established reference standards, or recommendations based on physiological needs.

Note: May not be appropriate nutrition diagnosis when weight gain is desired.

Etiology (Cause/Contributing Risk Factors)
Factors gathered during the nutrition assessment process that contribute to the existence or the maintenance of pathophysiological, psychosocial, situational, developmental, cultural, and/or environmental problems:

- Unsupported beliefs/attitudes about food, nutrition, and nutrition-related topics
- Food-and nutrition-related knowledge deficit concerning energy intake
- Lack of or limited access to healthful food choices, e.g., healthful food choices not provided as an option by caregiver or parent, homeless
- Lack of value for behavior change, competing values
- Medications that increase appetite, e.g., steroids, antidepressants
- Overfeeding of parenteral/enteral nutrition (PN/EN)
- Calories/kcal/kJ unaccounted for from IV infusion and/or medications
- Unwilling or disinterested in reducing energy intake
- Failure to adjust for lifestyle changes and decreased metabolism (e.g., aging)
- Failure to adjust for restricted mobility due to recovery from injury, surgical procedure, other
- Resolution of prior hypermetabolism without reduction in intake

Signs/Symptoms (Defining Characteristics)
A typical cluster of subjective and objective signs and symptoms gathered during the nutrition assessment process that provide evidence that a problem exists; quantify the problem and describe its severity.

Nutrition Assessment Category	Potential Indicators of This Nutrition Diagnosis (one or more must be present)
Biochemical Data, Medical Tests and Procedures	• Abnormal liver function tests after prolonged exposure (3 to 6 weeks) • ↑ Respiratory quotient >1.0
Anthropometric Measurements	• Body fat percentage > 25% for men and > 32% for women • BMI > 25 (adults); BMI > 95th percentile (pediatrics) • Weight gain
Nutrition-Focused Physical Findings	• Increased body adiposity • Increased respiratory rate

Arrows used with laboratory values: ↑ represents above reference standard and ↓ represents below reference standard.

Excessive Energy Intake (NI-1.3)

Food/Nutrition-Related History	Reports or observations of: • Intake of energy in excess of estimated or measured energy needs • Intake of high caloric density or large portions of foods/beverages • EN/PN more than estimated or measured (e.g., indirect calorimetry) energy expenditure
Client History	

Updated: 2013 Edition

DIAGNOSIS

Predicted Suboptimal Energy Intake (NI-1.4)

Definition

Future energy intake that is anticipated, based on observation, experience, or scientific reason, to be less than estimated energy expenditure, established reference standards, or recommendations based on physiological needs.

Note: May not be an appropriate nutrition diagnosis during weight loss. Use Inadequate Energy Intake (NI-1.2) when current energy intake is less than energy expenditure.

Etiology (Cause/Contributing Risk Factors)

Factors gathered during the nutrition assessment process that contribute to the existence or the maintenance of pathophysiological, psychosocial, situational, developmental, cultural, and/or environmental problems:

- Scheduled or planned procedure or medical therapy that is predicted to increase energy requirements
- Scheduled or planned medical therapy or medication that is predicted to decrease ability to consume sufficient energy
- Anticipated change in physical demands of work or leisure activities (e.g., job change, training for competitive sports)
- Stressful life event or living situation (e.g., death in family, divorce, loss of home) that, in the past, resulted in suboptimal energy intake

Signs/Symptoms (Defining Characteristics)

A typical cluster of subjective and objective signs and symptoms gathered during the nutrition assessment process that provide evidence that a problem exists; quantify the problem and describe its severity.

Nutrition Assessment Category	Potential Indicators of This Nutrition Diagnosis (one or more must be present)
Biochemical Data, Medical Tests and Procedures	
Anthropometric Measurements	• Population-based anthropometric data indicating suboptimal energy intake
Nutrition-Focused Physical Findings	• Population-based data on acute and chronic disease prevalence indicating suboptimal energy intake

Predicted Suboptimal Energy Intake (NI-1.4)

Food/Nutrition-Related History	Reports or observations of: • Estimated energy intake from all sources less than projected needs • History of marginal or suboptimal energy intake • Projected change in ability to shop, prepare, and/or consume sufficient energy • Medications that are anticipated to decrease appetite or affect ability to consume sufficient energy • No prior knowledge of need for food- and nutrition-related recommendations • Projected increase in level of physical activity
Client History	• Scheduled procedure or therapy known to increase energy need or change ability to consume sufficient energy • History or presence of a condition for which research shows an increased incidence of increased energy expenditure • History or presence of a condition for which research shows an increased incidence of suboptimal energy intake • Client report of recent or anticipated life stress or change

Updated: 2013 Edition

DIAGNOSIS

Predicted Excessive Energy Intake (NI-1.5)

Definition

Future energy intake that is anticipated, based on observation, experience, or scientific reason, to exceed estimated energy expenditure, established reference standards, or recommendations based on physiological needs.

Note: May not be appropriate nutrition diagnosis when weight gain is desired. Use Excessive Energy Intake (NI-1.3) when current energy intake is more than energy expenditure.

Etiology (Cause/Contributing Risk Factors)

Factors gathered during the nutrition assessment process that contribute to the existence or the maintenance of pathophysiological, psychosocial, situational, developmental, cultural, and/or environmental problems:

- Anticipated change in physical demands with periods of immobility or reduced physical activity
- Family or social history or culture of overeating
- Genetic predisposition to overweight/obesity
- Physiological condition associated with altered metabolism
- Scheduled or planned medical therapy or medication that is predicted to reduce metabolic rate/metabolism
- Stressful life event or living situation (e.g., death in family, divorce, loss of home) that, in the past, resulted in excessive energy intake

Signs/Symptoms (Defining Characteristics)

A typical cluster of subjective and objective signs and symptoms gathered during the nutrition assessment process that provide evidence that a problem exists; quantify the problem and describe its severity.

Nutrition Assessment Category	Potential Indicators of This Nutrition Diagnosis (one or more must be present)
Biochemical Data, Medical Tests and Procedures	
Anthropometric Measurements	• Population-based anthropometric data indicating excessive energy intake
Nutrition-Focused Physical Findings	• Population-based data on acute and chronic disease prevalence indicating excessive energy intake

Predicted Excessive Energy Intake (NI-1.5)

Food/Nutrition-Related History	Reports or observations of: • Estimated energy intake from all sources more than projected needs at new lower metabolic level • Estimated energy intake from all sources more than projected needs at new lower physical activity level • History of excessive energy intake at previous metabolic level • History of excessive energy intake at previous physical activity level • Recent or planned change in mobility and/or ability to engage in physical activity • Projected change in ability to shop and/or prepare food • Medications that increase appetite • Recent or planned change in physical activity • No prior knowledge of need for food- and nutrition-related recommendations
Client History	• Scheduled surgical procedure or medical therapy known to decrease energy need • History or presence of a condition for which research shows an increased incidence of decreased energy expenditure • History or presence of a condition for which research shows an increased incidence of excessive energy intake

DIAGNOSIS

Updated: 2013 Edition

Inadequate* Oral Intake (NI-2.1)

Definition
Oral food/beverage intake that is less than established reference standards or recommendations based on physiological needs.

> Note:This nutrition diagnosis does not include intake via oroenteric tube.
>
> May not be an appropriate nutrition diagnosis when the goal is weight loss, during end-of-life care, upon initiation of feeding, or during combined oral/EN/PN therapy.
>
> Whenever possible, nutrient intake data should be considered in combination with clinical, biochemical, anthropometric information, medical diagnosis, clinical status, and/or other factors as well as diet to provide a valid assessment of nutritional status based on a totality of the evidence. (Institute of Medicine. Dietary Reference Intakes: Applications in Dietary Assessment. Washington, DC: National Academies Press; 2000.)

Etiology (Cause/Contributing Risk Factors)
Factors gathered during the nutrition assessment process that contribute to the existence or the maintenance of pathophysiological, psychosocial, situational, developmental, cultural, and/or environmental problems:

- Physiological causes increasing nutrient needs, e.g., due to prolonged catabolic illness
- Decreased ability to consume sufficient energy, e.g., increased nutrient needs due to prolonged catabolic illness
- Lack of or limited access to food, e.g., economic constraints, restricting food given to elderly and/or children
- Limited food acceptance due to physiological or behavioral issues, aversion, or unsupported beliefs/attitudes
- Cultural practices that affect ability to access food
- Food- and nutrition-related knowledge deficit concerning appropriate oral food/beverage intake
- Psychological causes such as depression and disordered eating

Signs/Symptoms (Defining Characteristics)
A typical cluster of subjective and objective signs and symptoms gathered during the nutrition assessment process that provide evidence that a problem exists; quantify the problem and describe its severity.

Nutrition Assessment Category	Potential Indicators of This Nutrition Diagnosis (one or more must be present)
Biochemical Data, Medical Tests and Procedures	
Anthropometric Measurements	• Weight loss, insufficient growth velocity

*If a synonym for the term "inadequate" is helpful or needed, an approved alternate is the word "suboptimal."

Inadequate* Oral Intake (NI-2.1)

Nutrition-Focused Physical Findings	• Dry skin, mucous membranes, poor skin turgor • Anorexia, nausea, or vomiting • Change in appetite or taste • Clinical evidence of vitamin/mineral deficiency
Food/Nutrition-Related History	Reports or observations of: • Estimates of insufficient intake of energy or high-quality protein from diet when compared to requirements • Economic constraints that limit food availability • Excessive consumption of alcohol or other drugs that reduce hunger • Medications that cause anorexia • Limited food/beverage intake inconsistent with nutrition reference standards for type, variety, diet quality • less than optimal reliance on foods, food groups, supplements or nutrition support
Client History	• Conditions associated with a diagnosis or treatment of catabolic illness such as AIDS, tuberculosis, anorexia nervosa, sepsis or infection from recent surgery, depression, acute or chronic pain • Protein and/or nutrient malabsorption

DIAGNOSIS

Updated: 2011 Edition

*If a synonym for the term "inadequate" is helpful or needed, an approved alternate is the word "suboptimal."

4th Edition

Excessive Oral Intake (NI-2.2)

Definition
Oral food/beverage intake that exceeds estimated energy needs, established reference standards, or recommendations based on physiological needs.

> *Note: This nutrition diagnosis does not include intake via oroenteric tube.*
> *May not be an appropriate nutrition diagnosis when weight gain is desired.*

Etiology (Cause/Contributing Risk Factors)
Factors gathered during the nutrition assessment process that contribute to the existence or the maintenance of pathophysiological, psychosocial, situational, developmental, cultural, and/or environmental problems:

- Unsupported beliefs/attitudes about food, nutrition, and nutrition-related topics
- Food- and nutrition-related knowledge deficit concerning appropriate oral food/beverage intake
- Lack of or limited access to healthful food choices, e.g., healthful food choices not provided as an option by caregiver or parent, homeless
- Lack of value for behavior change, competing values
- Inability to limit or refuse offered foods
- Lack of food planning, purchasing, and preparation skills
- Loss of appetite awareness
- Medications that increase appetite, e.g., steroids, antidepressants
- Psychological causes such as depression and disordered eating
- Unwilling or disinterested in reducing intake

Signs/Symptoms (Defining Characteristics)
A typical cluster of subjective and objective signs and symptoms gathered during the nutrition assessment process that provide evidence that a problem exists; quantify the problem and describe its severity.

Nutrition Assessment Category	Potential Indicators of This Nutrition Diagnosis (one or more must be present)
Biochemical Data, Medical Tests and Procedures	
Anthropometric Measurements	• Weight gain not attributed to fluid retention or normal growth
Nutrition-Focused Physical Findings	

DIAGNOSIS

Excessive Oral Intake (NI-2.2)

Food/Nutrition-Related History	Reports or observations of: • Intake of high caloric-density foods/beverages (juice, soda, or alcohol) at meals and/or snacks • Intake of large portions of foods/beverages, food groups, or specific food items • Estimated intake that exceeds estimated or measured energy needs • Highly variable estimated daily energy intake • Binge eating patterns • Frequent, excessive fast food or restaurant intake
Client History	• Conditions associated with a diagnosis or treatment, e.g., obesity, overweight, or metabolic syndrome, depression, anxiety disorder

Updated: 2011 Edition

DIAGNOSIS

Inadequate* Enteral Nutrition Infusion (NI-2.3)

Definition

Enteral infusion that provides fewer calories/kcal/kJ or nutrients compared to established reference standards or recommendations based on physiological needs.

> *Note: May not be an appropriate nutrition diagnosis when recommendation is for weight loss, during end-of-life care, upon initiation of feeding, or during acute stressed states (e.g., surgery, organ failure).*
>
> *Whenever possible, nutrient intake data should be considered in combination with clinical, biochemical, anthropometric information, medical diagnosis, clinical status, and/or other factors as well as diet to provide a valid assessment of nutritional status based on a totality of the evidence. (Institute of Medicine. Dietary Reference Intakes: Applications in Dietary Assessment. Washington, DC: National Academies Press; 2000.)*

Etiology (Cause/Contributing Risk Factors)

Factors gathered during the nutrition assessment process that contribute to the existence or the maintenance of pathophysiological, psychosocial, situational, developmental, cultural, and/or environmental problems:

- Altered absorption or metabolism of nutrients, e.g., medications
- Food- and nutrition-related knowledge deficit concerning appropriate formula/formulation given for EN
- Lack of, compromised, or incorrect access for delivering EN
- Physiological causes increasing nutrient needs, e.g., due to accelerated growth, wound healing, chronic infection, multiple fractures
- Intolerance of EN
- Infusion volume not reached or schedule for infusion interrupted

Signs/Symptoms (Defining Characteristics)

A typical cluster of subjective and objective signs and symptoms gathered during the nutrition assessment process that provide evidence that a problem exists; quantify the problem and describe its severity.

If a synonym for the term "inadequate" is helpful or needed, an approved alternate is the word "suboptimal."

Inadequate* Enteral Nutrition Infusion (NI-2.3)

Nutrition Assessment Category	Potential Indicators of This Nutrition Diagnosis (one or more must be present)
Biochemical Data, Medical Tests and Procedures	• ↓ Metabolic cart/indirect calorimetry measurement, e.g., respiratory quotient < 0.7 • Vitamin/mineral abnormalities: ◦ ↓ Calcium < 9.2 mg/dL (2.3 mmol/L) ◦ Vitamin K—abnormal international normalized ratio (INR) ◦ ↓ Copper < 70 μg/dL (11 μmol/L) ◦ ↓ Zinc < 78 μg/dL (12 μmol/L) ◦ ↓ Iron < 50 μg/dL(nmol/L); iron-binding capacity < 250 μg/dL (44.8 μmol/L)
Anthropometric Measurements	• Growth failure, based on reference growth standards, e.g. National Center for Health Statistics (NCHS) and fetal growth failure • Insufficient maternal weight gain • Lack of planned weight gain • Unintentional weight loss of ≥ 5% in 1 month or ≥ 10% in 6 months (not attributed to fluid) in adults • Any weight loss in infants or children • Underweight (BMI < 18.5)
Nutrition-Focused Physical Findings	• Clinical evidence of vitamin/mineral deficiency (e.g., hair loss, bleeding gums, pale nail beds, neurologic changes) • Evidence of dehydration, e.g., dry mucous membranes, poor skin turgor • Loss of skin integrity, delayed wound healing, or pressure ulcers • Loss of muscle mass and/or subcutaneous fat • Nausea, vomiting, diarrhea
Food/Nutrition-Related History	Reports or observations of: • Inadequate EN volume compared to estimated or measured (indirect calorimetry) requirements • Feeding tube in wrong position or removed • Altered capacity for desired levels of physical activity or exercise, easy fatigue with increased activity • Suboptimal feeding position
Client History	• Conditions associated with a diagnosis or treatment, e.g., intestinal resection, Crohn's disease, HIV/AIDS, burns, preterm birth, malnutrition

DIAGNOSIS

Arrows used with laboratory values: ↑ represents above reference standard and ↓ represents below reference standard.
Updated: 2011 Edition

*If a synonym for the term "inadequate" is helpful or needed, an approved alternate is the word "suboptimal."

Excessive Enteral Nutrition Infusion (NI-2.4)

Definition

Enteral infusion that provides more calories/kcal/kJ or nutrients compared to established reference standards or recommendations based on physiological needs.

Etiology (Cause/Contributing Risk Factors)

Factors gathered during the nutrition assessment process that contribute to the existence or the maintenance of pathophysiological, psychosocial, situational, developmental, cultural, and/or environmental problems:

- Physiological causes, e.g., decreased needs related to low activity levels with critical illness or organ failure
- Food- and nutrition-related knowledge deficit concerning appropriate amount of enteral nutrition

Signs/Symptoms (Defining Characteristics)

A typical cluster of subjective and objective signs and symptoms gathered during the nutrition assessment process that provide evidence that a problem exists; quantify the problem and describe its severity.

Nutrition Assessment Category	Potential Indicators of This Nutrition Diagnosis (one or more must be present)
Biochemical Data, Medical Tests and Procedures	• ↑ BUN:creatinine ratio (protein) • Hyperglycemia (carbohydrate) • Hypercapnia
Anthropometric Measurements	• Weight gain in excess of lean tissue accretion
Nutrition-Focused Physical Findings	• Edema with excess fluid administration
Food/Nutrition-Related History	Reports or observations of: • Estimated intake from enteral nutrients that is consistently more than recommended intake for carbohydrate, protein, and fat • Use of drugs that reduce requirements or impair metabolism of energy, protein, fat, or fluid. • Unrealistic expectations of weight gain or ideal weight
Client History	

Arrows used with laboratory values: ↑ represents above reference standard and ↓ represents below reference standard.

Updated: 2011 Edition

Less than Optimal Enteral Nutrition Composition or Modality (NI-2.5)

Definition
Enteral nutrition composition (nutrient components) or modality (delivery and administration) that is inconsistent with evidence-based practice.

Etiology (Cause/Contributing Risk Factors)
Factors gathered during the nutrition assessment process that contribute to the existence or the maintenance of pathophysiological, psychosocial, situational, developmental, cultural, and/or environmental problems:

- Physiological causes, e.g., improvement in patient/client status, allowing return to total or partial oral diet; changes in the course of disease resulting in changes in feeding and/or nutrient requirements
- Food and nutrition-related knowledge deficit concerning EN product
- End-of-life care if patient/client or family do not desire nutrition support

Signs/Symptoms (Defining Characteristics)
A typical cluster of subjective and objective signs and symptoms gathered during the nutrition assessment process that provide evidence that a problem exists; quantify the problem and describe its severity.

Nutrition Assessment Category	Potential Indicators of This Nutrition Diagnosis (one or more must be present)
Biochemical Data, Medical Tests and Procedures	• Abnormal levels of markers specific for various nutrients, e.g., hyperphosphatemia in patient/client receiving feedings with a high phosphorus content, hypokalemia in patient/client receiving feedings with low potassium content
Anthropometric Measurements	• Weight gain in excess of lean tissue accretion • Weight loss
Nutrition-Focused Physical Findings	• Edema with excess fluid administration • Loss of subcutaneous fat and muscle stores • Nausea, vomiting, diarrhea, high gastric residual volume

DIAGNOSIS

4th Edition

Less than Optimal Enteral Nutrition Composition or Modality (NI-2.5)

Food/Nutrition-Related History	Reports or observations of: • Estimated intake from enteral nutrients that is consistently more or less than recommended intake for carbohydrate, protein, and/or fat– especially related to patient/client's ability to consume an oral diet that meets needs at this point in time • Estimated intake of other nutrients that is consistently more or less than recommended • Formula composition or type that is inconsistent with evidence-based practice • Verbalizations or written responses that are inaccurate or incomplete • History of enteral or parenteral nutrition intolerance
Client History	• Resolving or improved GI function • Conditions associated with a diagnosis or treatment, e.g., major elective surgery, trauma, burns, head and neck cancer, and critically ill patients, acute lung injury, acute respiratory distress syndrome, treatments/therapy requiring interruption of infusion, transfer of nutrition care to a new setting or level of care, end-of-life care

Updated: 2013 Edition

Inadequate* Parenteral Nutrition Infusion (NI-2.6)

Definition

Parenteral infusion that provides fewer calories/kcal/kJ or nutrients compared to established reference standards or recommendations based on physiological needs.

> *Note: May not be an appropriate nutrition diagnosis when recommendation is for weight loss, during end-of-life care, upon initiation of feeding, or during acute stressed states (e.g., surgery, organ failure).*
>
> *Whenever possible, nutrient intake data should be considered in combination with clinical, biochemical, anthropometric information, medical diagnosis, clinical status, and/or other factors as well as diet to provide a valid assessment of nutritional status based on a totality of the evidence. (Institute of Medicine. Dietary Reference Intakes: Applications in Dietary Assessment. Washington, DC: National Academies Press; 2000.)*

Etiology (Cause/Contributing Risk Factors)

Factors gathered during the nutrition assessment process that contribute to the existence or the maintenance of pathophysiological, psychosocial, situational, developmental, cultural, and/or environmental problems:

- Altered absorption or metabolism of nutrients, e.g., medications
- Food- and nutrition-related knowledge deficit concerning appropriate formula/ formulation given for PN
- Lack of, compromised, or incorrect access for delivering PN
- Physiological causes increasing nutrient needs, e.g., due to accelerated growth, wound healing, chronic infection, multiple fractures
- Intolerance of PN
- Infusion volume not reached or schedule for infusion interrupted

Signs/Symptoms (Defining Characteristics)

A typical cluster of subjective and objective signs and symptoms gathered during the nutrition assessment process that provide evidence that a problem exists; quantify the problem and describe its severity.

If a synonym for the term "inadequate" is helpful or needed, an approved alternate is the word "suboptimal."

4th Edition

DIAGNOSIS

Inadequate* Parenteral Nutrition Infusion (NI-2.6)

Nutrition Assessment Category	Potential Indicators of This Nutrition Diagnosis (one or more must be present)
Biochemical Data, Medical Tests and Procedures	• ↓ Metabolic cart/indirect calorimetry measurement, e.g., respiratory quotient < 0.7 • Vitamin/mineral abnormalities: ▪ ↓ Calcium < 9.2 mg/dL (2.3 mmol/L) ▪ Vitamin K—abnormal international normalized ratio (INR) ▪ ↓ Copper < 70 µg/dL (11 µmol/L) ▪ ↓ Zinc < 78 µg/dL (12 µmol/L) ▪ ↓ Iron < 50 µg/dL(nmol/L); iron-binding capacity < 250 µg/dL (44.8 µmol/L)
Anthropometric Measurements	• Growth failure, based on reference growth standards, e.g. National Center for Health Statistics (NCHS) and fetal growth failure • Insufficient maternal weight gain • Lack of planned weight gain • Unintentional weight loss of ≥ 5% in 1 month or ≥ 10% in 6 months (not attributed to fluid) in adults • Any weight loss in infants or children • Underweight (BMI < 18.5)
Nutrition-Focused Physical Findings	• Clinical evidence of vitamin/mineral deficiency (e.g., hair loss, bleeding gums, pale nail beds, neurologic changes) • Evidence of dehydration, e.g., dry mucous membranes, poor skin turgor • Loss of skin integrity, delayed wound healing, or pressure ulcers • Loss of muscle mass and/or subcutaneous fat • Nausea, vomiting, diarrhea
Food/Nutrition-Related History	Reports or observations of: • Inadequate PN volume compared to estimated or measured (indirect calorimetry) requirements • Feeding tube or venous access in wrong position or removed • Altered capacity for desired levels of physical activity or exercise, easy fatigue with increased activity
Client History	• Conditions associated with a diagnosis or treatment, e.g., intestinal resection, Crohn's disease, HIV/AIDS, burns, pre-term birth, malnutrition

Arrows used with laboratory values: ↑ *represents above reference standard and* ↓ *represents below reference standard*
Created: 2011 Edition
If a synonym for the term "inadequate" is helpful or needed, an approved alternate is the word "suboptimal."

Excessive Parenteral Nutrition Infusion (NI-2.7)

Definition
Parenteral infusion that provides more calories/kcal/kJ or nutrients compared to established reference standards or recommendations based on physiological needs.

Etiology (Cause/Contributing Risk Factors)
Factors gathered during the nutrition assessment process that contribute to the existence or the maintenance of pathophysiological, psychosocial, situational, developmental, cultural, and/or environmental problems:

- Physiological causes, e.g., decreased needs related to low activity levels with critical illness or organ failure
- Food- and nutrition-related knowledge deficit concerning appropriate amount of PN

Signs/Symptoms (Defining Characteristics)
A typical cluster of subjective and objective signs and symptoms gathered during the nutrition assessment process that provide evidence that a problem exists; quantify the problem and describe its severity.

Nutrition Assessment Category	Potential Indicators of This Nutrition Diagnosis (one or more must be present)
Biochemical Data, Medical Tests and Procedures	• ↑ BUN:creatinine ratio (protein) • Hyperglycemia (carbohydrate) • Hypercapnia • ↑ liver enzymes
Anthropometric Measurements	• Weight gain in excess of lean tissue accretion
Nutrition-Focused Physical Findings	• Edema with excess fluid administration
Food/Nutrition-Related History	Reports or observations of: • Estimated intake from parenteral nutrients that is consistently more than recommended intake for carbohydrate, protein, and fat • Use of drugs that reduce requirements or impair metabolism of energy, protein, fat, or fluid. • Unrealistic expectations of weight gain or ideal weight
Client History	

Arrows used with laboratory values: ↑ represents above reference standard and ↓ represents below reference standard.

Created: 2011 Edition

DIAGNOSIS

Less than Optimal Parenteral Nutrition Composition or Modality (NI-2.8)

Definition

Parenteral nutrition composition (nutrient components) or modality (delivery and administration) that is inconsistent with evidence-based practice.

Etiology (Cause/Contributing Risk Factors)

Factors gathered during the nutrition assessment process that contribute to the existence or the maintenance of pathophysiological, psychosocial, situational, developmental, cultural, and/or environmental problems:

- Physiological causes, e.g., improvement in patient/client status, allowing return to total or partial oral diet; changes in the course of disease resulting in changes in feeding and/or nutrient requirements
- Food and nutrition-related knowledge deficit concerning PN product
- End-of-life care if patient/client or family do not desire nutrition support

Signs/Symptoms (Defining Characteristics)

A typical cluster of subjective and objective signs and symptoms gathered during the nutrition assessment process that provide evidence that a problem exists; quantify the problem and describe its severity.

Nutrition Assessment Category	Potential Indicators of This Nutrition Diagnosis (one or more must be present)
Biochemical Data, Medical Tests and Procedures	• ↑ liver function tests in patient/client on long-term (more than 3 to 6 weeks) nutrition support • Abnormal levels of markers specific for various nutrients, e.g., hyperphosphatemia in patient/client receiving feedings with a high phosphorus content, hypokalemia in patient/client receiving feedings with low potassium content
Anthropometric Measurements	• Weight gain in excess of lean tissue accretion • Weight loss
Nutrition-Focused Physical Findings	• Edema with excess fluid administration • Loss of subcutaneous fat and muscle stores • Nausea

Arrows used with laboratory values: ↑ represents above reference standard and ↓ represents below reference standard.

Less than Optimal Parenteral Nutrition Composition or Modality (NI-2.8)

Food/Nutrition-Related History	Reports or observations of: • Estimated intake from parenteral nutrients that is consistently more or less than recommended intake for carbohydrate, protein, and/or fat—especially related to patient/client's ability to consume an oral diet that meets needs at this point in time • Estimated intake of other nutrients that is consistently more or less than recommended • Formula composition or type that is inconsistent with evidence-based practice • Verbalizations or written responses that are inaccurate or incomplete • History of enteral or parenteral nutrition intolerance
Client History	• Complications such as fatty liver in the absence of other causes • Resolving or improved GI function • Conditions associated with a diagnosis or treatment, e.g., major elective surgery, trauma, burns, head and neck cancer, and critically ill patients, acute lung injury, acute respiratory distress syndrome, treatments/therapy requiring interruption of infusion, transfer of nutrition care to a new setting or level of care, end-of-life care

Updated: 2013 Edition

DIAGNOSIS

Limited Food Acceptance (NI-2.9)

Definition
Oral food/beverage intake that is inconsistent with reference standard intake for type, variety, or quality.

> *Note: May not be an appropriate nutrition diagnosis for individuals with anorexia nervosa, bulimia nervosa, binge eating disorder, or eating disorder not otherwise specified (EDNOS). Please consider using Disordered Eating Pattern (NB-1.5).*

Etiology (Cause/Contributing Risk Factors)
Factors gathered during the nutrition assessment process that contribute to the existence or the maintenance of pathophysiological, psychosocial, situational, developmental, cultural, and/or environmental problems:

- Physiological causes, e.g., pain, discomfort, or functional issues in the GI tract, developmental delay, neurological disorders
- Aversion to food/beverages in mouth, throat, or hands
- Self-limitation of foods/food groups due to food preference
- Behavioral issues including caregiver issues and eating behavior that serves a purpose other than nourishment
- Unsupported beliefs and attitudes

Signs/Symptoms (Defining Characteristics)
A typical cluster of subjective and objective signs and symptoms gathered during the nutrition assessment process that provide evidence that a problem exists; quantify the problem and describe its severity.

Nutrition Assessment Category	Potential Indicators of This Nutrition Diagnosis (one or more must be present)
Biochemical Data, Medical Tests and Procedures	
Anthropometric Measurements	• Weight loss, insufficient growth velocity, weight gain due to reliance on low-variety or less than optimal intake
Nutrition-Focused Physical Findings	• Clinical evidence of vitamin/mineral deficiency • Erratic appetite
Food/Nutrition-Related History	Reports or observations of: • Limited food/beverage intake inconsistent with nutrition reference standards for type, variety, diet quality • Less than optimal reliance on foods, food groups, supplements, or nutrition support

Limited Food Acceptance (NI-2.9)

Client History	• Conditions associated with a diagnosis or treatment, e.g., developmental disabilities, sensory processing issues, autism, dental caries, long-term nutrition support, prematurity, neurological disorders, altered mental state, affected brain studies (MRI)

Updated: 2013 Edition

DIAGNOSIS

Inadequate* Fluid Intake (NI-3.1)

Definition
Lower intake of fluid-containing foods or substances compared to established reference standards or recommendations based on physiological needs.

> *Note: Whenever possible, nutrient intake data should be considered in combination with clinical, biochemical, anthropometric information, medical diagnosis, clinical status, and/or other factors as well as diet to provide a valid assessment of nutritional status based on a totality of the evidence. (Dietary Reference Intakes: Applications in Dietary Assessment. Institute of Medicine. Washington, D.C.: National Academies Press; 2000.)*

Etiology (Cause/Contributing Risk Factors)
Factors gathered during the nutrition assessment process that contribute to the existence or the maintenance of pathophysiological, psychosocial, situational, developmental, cultural, and/or environmental problems:

- Physiological causes increasing fluid needs due to climate/temperature change, increased exercise or conditions leading to increased fluid losses, fever causing increased insensible losses, decreased thirst sensation, or use of drugs that reduce thirst
- Lack of or limited access to fluid, e.g., economic constraints, unable to access fluid independently such as elderly or children
- Cultural practices that affect the ability to access fluid
- Food- and nutrition-related knowledge deficit concerning appropriate fluid intake
- Psychological causes, e.g., depression or disordered eating
- Impaired cognitive ability, including learning disabilities, neurological or sensory impairment, and/or dementia

Signs/Symptoms (Defining Characteristics)
A typical cluster of subjective and objective signs and symptoms gathered during the nutrition assessment process that provide evidence that a problem exists; quantify the problem and describe its severity.

Nutrition Assessment Category	Potential Indicators of This Nutrition Diagnosis (one or more must be present)
Biochemical Data, Medical Tests and Procedures	• Plasma or serum osmolality greater than 290 mOsm/kg • Abnormal BUN, Na • ↓ Urine volume • ↑ Urine specific gravity • Hyperglycemia in diabetic patient/client
Anthropometric Measurements	• Acute weight loss

Arrows used with laboratory values: ↑ represents above reference standard and ↓ represents below reference standard.

*If a synonym for the term "inadequate" is helpful or needed, an approved alternate is the word "suboptimal."

DIAGNOSIS

Inadequate* Fluid Intake (NI-3.1)

Nutrition-Focused Physical Findings	• Dry skin and mucous membranes, poor skin turgor, tachycardia and normal or hypotensive blood pressure, fever, increased respirations, flattened neck veins • Thirst • Difficulty swallowing • Increased insensible loss
Food/Nutrition-Related History	Reports or observations of: • Estimated intake of fluid less than requirements (e.g., per body surface area for pediatrics) • Use of drugs that reduce thirst
Client History	• Conditions associated with a diagnosis or treatment, e.g., dementia resulting in decreased recognition of thirst, dehydration, diabetes mellitus, alterations in renal function, diarrhea,vomiting, ileostomy, colostomy, infection

DIAGNOSIS

Updated: 2013 Edition

If a synonym for the term "inadequate" is helpful or needed, an approved alternate is the word "suboptimal."

Excessive Fluid Intake (NI-3.2)

Definition

Higher intake of fluid compared to established reference standards or recommendations based on physiological needs.

Etiology (Cause/Contributing Risk Factors)

Factors gathered during the nutrition assessment process that contribute to the existence or the maintenance of pathophysiological, psychosocial, situational, developmental, cultural, and/or environmental problems:

- Physiological causes, e.g., kidney, liver, cardiac, endocrine, neurological, and/or pulmonary dysfunction; diminished water and sodium losses due to changes in exercise or climate, syndrome of inappropriate antidiuretic hormone (SIADH)
- Food- and nutrition-related knowledge deficit concerning appropriate fluid intake
- Psychological causes such as depression and disordered eating

Signs/Symptoms (Defining Characteristics)

A typical cluster of subjective and objective signs and symptoms gathered during the nutrition assessment process that provide evidence that a problem exists; quantify the problem and describe its severity.

Nutrition Assessment Category	Potential Indicators of This Nutrition Diagnosis (one or more must be present)
Biochemical Data, Medical Tests and Procedures	• ↓ Plasma osmolality (270-280 mOsm/kg), only if positive fluid balance is in excess of positive sodium balance • ↓ Serum sodium in SIADH • ↓ Urine specific gravity
Anthropometric Measurements	• Weight gain
Nutrition-Focused Physical Findings	• Edema in the skin of the legs, sacral area, or diffusely; weeping of fluids from lower legs • Ascites • Pulmonary edema as evidenced by shortness of breath; orthopnea; crackles or rales • Nausea, vomiting, anorexia, headache, muscle spasms, convulsions • Shortness of breath or dyspnea with exertion or at rest • Providing medications in large amounts of fluid • Use of drugs that impair fluid excretion

Arrows used with laboratory values: ↑ represents above reference standard and ↓ represents below reference standard

Excessive Fluid Intake (NI-3.2)

Food/Nutrition-Related History	Reports or observations of: • Estimated intake of fluid more than requirements (e.g., per body surface area for pediatrics) • Estimated salt intake in excess of recommendations
Client History	• Conditions associated with a diagnosis or treatment, e.g., end-stage renal disease, nephrotic syndrome, heart failure, or liver disease • Coma (SIADH)

Updated: 2013 Edition

DIAGNOSIS

Suboptimal Bioactive Substance Intake (specify) (NI-4.1)

Definition
Lower intake of bioactive substances compared to established reference standards or recommendations based on physiological needs.

> *Note: Bioactive substances are not part of the Dietary Reference Intakes, and therefore there are no established minimum requirements or Tolerable Upper Intake Levels. However, food and nutrition professionals can assess whether estimated intakes are adequate or excessive using the patient/client goal or nutrition prescription for comparison.*
>
> *Working definition of bioactive substances—physiologically active components of foods that may have an effect on health. There is no scientific consensus about a definition for bioactive substances/components.*

Etiology (Cause/Contributing Risk Factors)
Factors gathered during the nutrition assessment process that contribute to the existence or the maintenance of pathophysiological, psychosocial, situational, developmental, cultural, and/or environmental problems:

- Food- and nutrition-related knowledge deficit concerning recommended bioactive substance intake
- Lack of or limited access to food that contains a bioactive substance
- Alteration in gastrointestinal tract structure and/or function

Signs/Symptoms (Defining Characteristics)
A typical cluster of subjective and objective signs and symptoms gathered during the nutrition assessment process that provide evidence that a problem exists; quantify the problem and describe its severity.

Nutrition Assessment Category	Potential Indicators of This Nutrition Diagnosis (one or more must be present)
Biochemical Data, Medical Tests and Procedures	
Anthropometric Measurements	
Nutrition-Focused Physical Findings	

Suboptimal Bioactive Substance Intake (specify) (NI-4.1)

Food/Nutrition-Related History	Reports or observations of: • Estimated intake of plant foods containing the following lower than recommended: • Soluble fiber, e.g., psyllium ($\downarrow$ total and LDL cholesterol) • Soy protein ($\downarrow$ total and LDL cholesterol) • β-glucan, e.g., whole oat products ($\downarrow$ total and LDL cholesterol) • Plant sterol and stanol esters, e.g., fortified margarines ($\downarrow$ total and LDL cholesterol) • Other substances (for which scientific evidence exists and a recommended intake level has been established) • Verbalizes inaccurate or incomplete knowledge about bioactive substances
Client History	• Conditions associated with a diagnosis or treatment, e.g., cardiovascular disease, elevated cholesterol

DIAGNOSIS

Updated: 2013 Edition

Excessive Bioactive Substance Intake (specify) (NI-4.2)

Definition

Higher intake of bioactive substances compared to established reference standards or recommendations based on physiological needs.

> Note: Bioactive substances are not part of the Dietary Reference Intakes, and therefore there are no established minimum requirements or Tolerable Upper Intake Levels. However, food and nutrition professionals can assess whether estimated intakes are adequate or excessive using the patient/client goal or nutrition prescription for comparison.
>
> Working definition of bioactive substances—physiologically active components of foods that may have an effect on health. There is no scientific consensus about a definition for bioactive substances/components.

Etiology (Cause/Contributing Risk Factors)

Factors gathered during the nutrition assessment process that contribute to the existence or the maintenance of pathophysiological, psychosocial, situational, developmental, cultural, and/or environmental problems:

- Food- and nutrition-related knowledge deficit concerning recommended bioactive substance intake including food additives
- Contamination, misname, mislabel or lack of labeling, misuse, recent brand change, recent dose increase, recent formulation change of substance consumed
- Frequent intake of foods containing bioactive substances
- Alteration in gastrointestinal tract structure and/or function
- Lack of or limited access to appropriate foods, e.g., inadequate markets with labeled food

Signs/Symptoms (Defining Characteristics)

A typical cluster of subjective and objective signs and symptoms gathered during the nutrition assessment process that provide evidence that a problem exists; quantify the problem and describe its severity.

Nutrition Assessment Category	Potential Indicators of This Nutrition Diagnosis (one or more must be present)
Biochemical Data, Medical Tests and Procedures	• Lab values indicating excessive intake of the specific substance, such as rapid ↓ in cholesterol from intake of stanol or sterol esters and a statin drug and related dietary changes or medications • ↑ Hepatic enzyme reflecting hepatocellular damage
Anthropometric Measurements	• Weight loss as a result of malabsorption or maldigestion

Arrows used with laboratory values: ↑ represents above reference standard and ↓ represents below reference standard

Excessive Bioactive Substance Intake (specify) (NI-4.2)

Nutrition-Focused Physical Findings	• Constipation, diarrhea, nausea, stomach pain, gas, cramps or bloating, vomiting, heartburn • Neurologic changes, e.g., anxiety, mental status changes • Cardiovascular changes, e.g., heart rate, blood pressure • Discomfort or pain associated with intake of foods rich in bioactive substances, e.g., soluble fiber, β-glucan, soy protein • Headache/migraine • Hives, flushing • Irritability or nervousness
Food/Nutrition-Related History	Reports or observations of: • High intake of plant foods containing: • Soy protein ($\downarrow$ total and LDL cholesterol) • β-glucan, e.g., whole oat products ($\downarrow$ total and LDL cholesterol) • Plant sterol and stanol esters, e.g., fortified margarines ($\downarrow$ total and LDL cholesterol) or other foods based on dietary substance, concentrate, metabolite, constituent, extract, or combination • Substances that interfere with digestion or absorption of foodstuffs • Ready access to available foods/products with bioactive substance, e.g., as from dietary supplement vendors • Attempts to use supplements or bioactive substances for weight loss, to treat constipation, or to prevent or cure chronic or acute disease • Other substances (for which scientific evidence exists and a recommended intake level has been established) • Intake of food additives for which patient/client is intolerant, e.g., yellow 5, yellow 6, safrole, FD&C Red #4, carmine, MSG, sulfites • Verbalizes inaccurate or incomplete knowledge about bioactive substances
Client History	• Conditions associated with a diagnosis or treatment, e.g., cardiovascular disease, elevated cholesterol, hypertension, asthma • Cardiovascular changes, e.g., EKG changes

DIAGNOSIS

rrows used with laboratory values: $\uparrow$ represents above reference standard and $\downarrow$ represents below reference standard.

Updated: 2013 Edition

4th Edition

Excessive Alcohol Intake (NI-4.3)

Definition
Intake more than the suggested limits for alcohol.

Etiology (Cause/Contributing Risk Factors)
Factors gathered during the nutrition assessment process that contribute to the existence or the maintenance of pathophysiological, psychosocial, situational, developmental, cultural, and/or environmental problems:

- Unsupported beliefs/attitudes about food, nutrition, and nutrition-related topics
- Food- and nutrition-related knowledge deficit concerning appropriate alcohol intake
- Lack of value for behavior change, competing values
- Alcohol addiction

Signs/Symptoms (Defining Characteristics)
A typical cluster of subjective and objective signs and symptoms gathered during the nutrition assessment process that provide evidence that a problem exists; quantify the problem and describe its severity.

Nutrition Assessment Category	Potential Indicators of This Nutrition Diagnosis (one or more must be present)
Biochemical Data, Medical Tests and Procedures	• ↑ aspartate aminotransferase (AST), gamma-glutamyl transferase (GGT), carbohydrate-deficient transferrin, mean corpuscular volume, blood alcohol levels
Anthropometric Measurements	
Nutrition-Focused Physical Findings	
Food/Nutrition-Related History	Reports or observations of: • Intake of > 2 drinks*/day (men) • Intake of > 1 drink*/day (women) • Binge drinking • Consumption of any alcohol when contraindicated, e.g., during pregnancy *1 drink = 5 oz (150 mL) wine, 12 oz (350 mL) beer, 1.5 oz (45 mL) distilled alcohol

Arrows used with laboratory values: ↑ represents above reference standard and ↓ represents below reference standard.

Excessive Alcohol Intake (NI-4.3)

Client History	• Conditions associated with a diagnosis or treatment, e.g., severe hypertri-glyceridemia, elevated blood pressure, depression, liver disease, pancreatitis • New medical diagnosis or change in existing diagnosis or condition • History of estimated alcohol intake in excess of recommended • Giving birth to an infant with fetal alcohol syndrome

Updated: 2013 Edition

DIAGNOSIS

4th Edition

Increased Nutrient Needs (Specify) (NI-5.1)

Definition

Increased need for a specific nutrient compared to established reference standards or recommendations based on physiological needs.

Etiology (Cause/Contributing Risk Factors)

Factors gathered during the nutrition assessment process that contribute to the existence or the maintenance of pathophysiological, psychosocial, situational, developmental, cultural, and/or environmental problems:

- Altered absorption or metabolism of nutrient, e.g., from medications
- Compromise of organs related to GI function, e.g., pancreas, liver
- Decreased functional length of intestine, e.g., short-bowel syndrome
- Decreased or compromised function of intestine, e.g., celiac disease, Crohn's disease
- Increased demand for nutrient, e.g., accelerated growth, wound healing, chronic infection

Signs/Symptoms (Defining Characteristics)

A typical cluster of subjective and objective signs and symptoms gathered during the nutrition assessment process that provide evidence that a problem exists; quantify the problem and describe its severity.

Nutrition Assessment Category	Potential Indicators of This Nutrition Diagnosis (one or more must be present)
Biochemical Data, Medical Tests and Procedures	• ↓ total cholesterol < 160 mg/dL, albumin, prealbumin, C-reactive protein, indicating increased stress and increased metabolic needs • Electrolyte/mineral (e.g., potassium, magnesium, phosphorus) abnormalities • Urinary or fecal losses of specific or related nutrient (e.g., fecal fat, d-xylose test) • Vitamin and/or mineral deficiency
Anthropometric Measurements	• Growth failure, based on reference growth standards , e.g. National Center for Health Statistics (NCHS) and fetal growth failure • Unintentional weight loss of ≥5% in 1 month or ≥10% in 6 months • Underweight (BMI < 18.5) • Low percent body fat and muscle mass

Arrows used with laboratory values: ↑ represents above reference standard and ↓ represents below reference standard

Increased Nutrient Needs (Specify) (NI-5.1)

Nutrition-Focused Physical Findings	• Clinical evidence of vitamin/mineral deficiency (e.g., hair loss, bleeding gums, pale nail beds) • Loss of skin integrity, delayed wound healing, or pressure ulcers • Loss of muscle mass, subcutaneous fat
Food/Nutrition-Related History	Reports or observations of: • Estimated intake of foods/supplements containing needed nutrient less than estimated requirements • Intake of foods that do not contain sufficient quantities of available nutrient (e.g., overprocessed, overcooked, or stored improperly) • Food- and nutrition-related knowledge deficit (e.g., lack of information, incorrect information or noncompliance with intake of needed nutrient) • Medications affecting absorption or metabolism of needed nutrient • Athletes or active individuals engaged in intense physical activity
Client History	• Conditions associated with a diagnosis or treatment, e.g., intestinal resection, Crohn's disease, HIV/AIDS, burns, pre-term birth, malnutrition

DIAGNOSIS

Updated: 2011 Edition

4th Edition

Malnutrition (NI-5.2)

Definition

Inadequate intake of protein and/or energy over prolonged periods of time resulting in loss of fat stores and/or muscle stores including starvation-related malnutrition, chronic disease or condition-related malnutrition and acute disease or injury-related malnutrition.

> *Note. The Academy and ASPEN continue to work with the National Center for Health Statistics to revise projected ICD-10 coding terminology to incorporate an etiology-based approach to malnutrition diagnosis (J Parenter Enteral Nutr. 2010;34(2):156-159). The Academy/ASPEN collaboration is in the process of developing characteristics to diagnose pediatric (ages 1-18) malnutrition.*
>
> *^The Academy/ASPEN recommend a minimum of two clinical characteristics or indicators be present for diagnosis of malnutrition in adults. For additional information, visit the Academy's Web page at: http://www.eatright.org/coverage.*

Etiology (Cause/Contributing Risk Factors)

Factors gathered during the nutrition assessment process that contribute to the existence or the maintenance of pathophysiological, psychosocial, situational, developmental, cultural, and/or environmental problems:

- Physiological causes increasing nutrient needs due to illness, acute or chronic or injury/trauma
- Alteration in gastrointestinal tract structure and/or function
- Lack of or limited access to food, e.g., economic constraints, restricting food given to elderly and/or children, neglect or abuse
- Cultural or religious practices that affect the ability to access food
- Food- and nutrition-related knowledge deficit concerning amount of energy and amount and type of dietary protein
- Psychological causes, e.g., depression or eating disorders

Signs/Symptoms (Defining Characteristics)

A typical cluster of subjective and objective signs and symptoms gathered during the nutrition assessment process that provide evidence that a problem exists; quantify the problem and describe its severity.

Nutrition Assessment Category	Potential Indicators of This Nutrition Diagnosis (one or more must be present)
Biochemical Data, Medical Tests and Procedures	*

* *In the past, hepatic transport protein measures (e.g. albumin and prealbumin) were used as indicators of malnutrition. See the Evidence Analysis Library questions on this topic at https://www. andevidencelibrary.com/topic. cfm?cat=4302*

Malnutrition (NI-5.2)

Anthropometric Measurements	• Malnutrition can occur at any weight/BMI • BMI < 18.5 indicates underweight; BMI for older adults (older than 65 years) < 22; BMI < 5th percentile in children • Failure to thrive, e.g., failure to attain desirable growth rates or developmental delay • Inadequate maternal weight gain • ^ Unintentional weight loss, adults, of > 20% in 1 year; > 10% in 6 months; > 7.5% in 3 months; > 5% in 1 month; or > 1 to 2% in 1 week • Growth, pediatrics, not gaining weight as expected and/or a shift downward in their growth percentiles, crossing two or more percentiles on their growth charts • Underweight with loss of fat and/or muscle
Nutrition-Focused Physical Findings	• ^Loss of subcutaneous fat, e.g., orbital, triceps, fat overlying the ribs • ^Muscle loss, e.g., wasting of the temples (temporalis muscle), clavicles (pectoralis & deltoids), shoulders (deltoids), interosseous muscles, scapula (latissimus dorsi, trapezious, deltoids), thigh (quadriceps) and calf (gastrocnemius) • ^Localized or generalized fluid accumulation (ex-tremities, vulvar/scrotal, acites) • Change in functional indicators, i.e., grip strength
Food/Nutrition-Related History	Reports or observations of: • ^Estimated energy intake < 50%-75% of estimated or measured RMR • Unable or unwilling to eat sufficient energy/protein to maintain a healthy weight • Food avoidance and/or lack of interest in food • Excessive consumption of alcohol or other drugs that reduce appetite • ^Change in functional indicators, e.g., grip strength or other measures of physical activity and/or strength

The Academy/ASPEN recommend a minimum of two clinical characteristics or indicators be present for diagnosis of
ialnutrition in adults. For additional information, visit the Academy's Web page at: http://www.eatright.org/coverage.

DIAGNOSIS

Malnutrition (NI-5.2)

Client History	Reports or observations of the following, for example: • Anorexia nervosa, benign esophageal stricture, abuse, neglect, poverty, frailty, and anything that results in limited access to food (associated with malnutrition in the context of environmental and social circumstances) • Organ failure, malignancies, rheumatoid diseases, gastrointestinal diseases, sarcopenic obesity, malabsorptive syndromes, and other etiologies including but not limited to diabetes, congestive heart failure, and chronic obstructive pulmonary disease (associated with malnutrition in the context of chronic disease/condition) • Major infections such as; sepsis, pneumonia, peritonitis, and wound infections, major burns, trauma, closed head injury, acute lung injury, adult respiratory distress syndrome, and selected major surgeries (associated with malnutrition in the context of acute injury/illness) • Existing medical diagnosis of malnutrition including malnutrition in the context of acute injury/illness, malnutrition in the context of chronic disease/condition and malnutrition in the context of environmental and social circumstances.

^ *The Academy/ASPEN recommend a minimum of two clinical characteristics or indicators be present for diagnosis of malnutrition in adults. For additional information, visit the Academy's Web page at: http://www.eatright.org/coverage.*

Updated: 2013 Edition

Inadequate* Protein–Energy Intake (NI-5.3)

Definition

Inadequate intake of protein and/or energy compared to established reference standards or recommendations based on physiological needs of short or recent duration.

> *Note: Whenever possible, nutrient intake data should be considered in combination with clinical, biochemical, anthropometric information, medical diagnosis, clinical status, and/ or other factors as well as diet to provide a valid assessment of nutritional status based on a totality of the evidence.* (Institute of Medicine. Dietary Reference Intakes: Applications in Dietary Assessment. *Washington, DC: National Academies Press; 2000.*)

Etiology (Cause/Contributing Risk Factors)

Factors gathered during the nutrition assessment process that contribute to the existence or the maintenance of pathophysiological, psychosocial, situational, developmental, cultural, and/or environmental problems:

- Physiological causes increasing nutrient needs due to catabolic illness, malabsorption
- Decreased ability to consume sufficient protein and/or energy
- Lack of or limited access to food, e.g., economic constraints, restricting food given or food selected
- Cultural or religious practices that affect ability to access food
- Food- and nutrition-related knowledge deficit concerning appropriate amount and type of dietary fat and/or protein
- Psychological causes such as depression and disordered eating

Signs/Symptoms (Defining Characteristics)

A typical cluster of subjective and objective signs and symptoms gathered during the nutrition assessment process that provide evidence that a problem exists; quantify the problem and describe its severity.

Nutrition Assessment Category	Potential Indicators of This Nutrition Diagnosis (one or more must be present)
Biochemical Data, Medical Tests and Procedures	• Normal albumin (in the setting of normal liver function despite decreased protein-energy intake)
Anthropometric Measurements	• Inadequate maternal weight gain (mild but not severe) • Weight loss of 7% in 3 months, >5% in 1 month, or 1% to 2% in 1 week in adults; any weight loss or failure to gain weight in children • Growth failure in children
Nutrition-Focused Physical Findings	• Slow wound healing in pressure ulcer or surgical patient/client

If a synonym for the term "inadequate" is helpful or needed, an approved alternate is the word "suboptimal."

4th Edition

DIAGNOSIS

Inadequate* Protein–Energy Intake (NI-5.3)

Food/Nutrition-Related History	Reports or observations of: • Estimated energy intake from diet less than estimated or measured RMR or recommended levels • Restriction or omission of food groups such as dairy or meat group foods (protein); bread or milk group foods (energy) • Recent food avoidance and/or lack of interest in food • Lack of ability to prepare meals • Excessive consumption of alcohol or other drugs that reduce hunger • Hunger in the face of inadequate access to food supply
Client History	• Conditions associated with a diagnosis or treatment of mild protein-energy malnutrition, recent illness (e.g., pulmonary or cardiac failure, flu, infection, surgery) • Nutrient malabsorption (e.g., bariatric surgery, diarrhea, steatorrhea) • Lack of funds for purchase of appropriate foods

Updated: 2011 Edition

If a synonym for the term "inadequate" is helpful or needed, an approved alternate is the word "suboptimal."

Decreased Nutrient Needs (Specify) (NI-5.4)

Definition

Decreased need for a specific nutrient compared to established reference standards or recommendations based on physiological needs.

Etiology (Cause/Contributing Risk Factors)

Factors gathered during the nutrition assessment process that contribute to the existence or the maintenance of pathophysiological, psychosocial, situational, developmental, cultural, and/or environmental problems:

- Renal dysfunction
- Liver dysfunction
- Altered cholesterol metabolism/regulation
- Heart failure
- Food intolerances, e.g., irritable bowel syndrome

Signs/Symptoms (Defining Characteristics)

A typical cluster of subjective and objective signs and symptoms gathered during the nutrition assessment process that provide evidence that a problem exists; quantify the problem and describe its severity.

Nutrition Assessment Category	Potential Indicators of This Nutrition Diagnosis (one or more must be present)
Biochemical Data, Medical Tests and Procedures	• ↑ Total cholesterol > 200 mg/dL (5.2 mmol/L), ↑ LDL cholesterol > 100 mg/dL (2.59 mmol/L), ↓ HDL cholesterol < 40 mg/dL (1.036 mmol/L), ↑ triglycerides > 150 mg/dL (1.695 mmol/L) • ↑ Phosphorus > 5.5 mg/dL (1.78 mmol/L) • ↓ Glomerular filtration rate (GFR) < 90 mL/min/1.73 m^2 • ↑ BUN, creatinine, potassium • ↑ Liver function tests indicating severe liver disease
Anthropometric Measurements	• Interdialytic weight gain greater than expected
Nutrition-Focused Physical Findings	• Edema/fluid retention
Food/Nutrition-Related History	Reports or observations of: • Estimated intake higher than recommended for fat, phosphorus, sodium, protein, fiber

Arrows used with laboratory values: ↑ *represents above reference standard and* ↓ *represents below reference standard.*

DIAGNOSIS

Decreased Nutrient Needs (Specify) (NI-5.4)

Client History	• Conditions associated with a diagnosis or treatment that require a specific type and/or amount of nutrient, e.g., cardiovascular disease (fat), early renal disease (protein, phos), ESRD (phos, sodium, potassium, fluid), advanced liver disease (protein), heart failure (sodium, fluid), irritable bowel disease/Crohn's flare up (fiber) • Diagnosis of hypertension, confusion related to liver disease

Imbalance of Nutrients (NI-5.5)

Definition

An undesirable combination of nutrients, such that the amount of one nutrient interferes with or alters absorption and/or utilization of another nutrient.

Etiology (Cause/Contributing Risk Factors)

Factors gathered during the nutrition assessment process that contribute to the existence or the maintenance of pathophysiological, psychosocial, situational, developmental, cultural, and/or environmental problems:

- Consumption of high-dose nutrient supplements
- Food- and nutrition-related knowledge deficit concerning nutrient interactions
- Unsupported beliefs/attitudes about food, nutrition, and nutrition-related information
- Food faddism
- Insufficient electrolyte replacement when initiating feeding (PN/EN, including oral)

Signs/Symptoms (Defining Characteristics)

A typical cluster of subjective and objective signs and symptoms gathered during the nutrition assessment process that provide evidence that a problem exists; quantify the problem and describe its severity.

Nutrition Assessment Category	Potential Indicators of This Nutrition Diagnosis (one or more must be present)
Biochemical Data, Medical Tests and Procedures	- Severe hypophosphatemia (in the presence of increased carbohydrate) - Severe hypokalemia (in the presence of increased protein) - Severe hypomagnesemia (in the presence of increased carbohydrate)
Anthropometric Data	
Nutrition-Focused Physical Findings	- Diarrhea or constipation (iron supplements) - Epigastric pain, nausea, vomiting, diarrhea (zinc supplements)
Food/Nutrition-Related History	Reports or observations of: - Estimated intake of iron supplements (decreased zinc absorption) higher than recommended - Estimated intake of zinc supplements (decreased copper status) higher than recommended - Estimated intake of manganese (decreased iron status) higher than recommended
Client History	- Refeeding syndrome

Updated: 2013 Edition

4th Edition

DIAGNOSIS

Inadequate* Fat Intake (NI-5.6.1)

Definition

Lower fat intake compared to established reference standards or recommendations based on physiological needs.

> Note: May not be an appropriate nutrition diagnosis when the goal is weight loss or during end-of-life care.
>
> Whenever possible, nutrient intake data should be considered in combination with clinical, biochemical, anthropometric information, medical diagnosis, clinical status, and/or other factors as well as diet to provide a valid assessment of nutritional status based on a totality of the evidence. (Dietary Reference Intakes: Applications in Dietary Assessment. Institute of Medicine. Washington, D.C.: National Academies Press; 2000).

Etiology (Cause/Contributing Risk Factors)

Factors gathered during the nutrition assessment process that contribute to the existence or the maintenance of pathophysiological, psychosocial, situational, developmental, cultural, and/or environmental problems:

- Alteration in gastrointestinal tract structure and/or function
- Less than optimal food choices, e.g., economic constraints, restricting food given to elderly and/or children, specific food choices
- Cultural practices that affect ability to make appropriate food choices
- Food- and nutrition-related knowledge deficit concerning appropriate amount of dietary fat
- Psychological causes such as depression and disordered eating

Signs/Symptoms (Defining Characteristics)

A typical cluster of subjective and objective signs and symptoms gathered during the nutrition assessment process that provide evidence that a problem exists; quantify the problem and describe its severity.

Nutrition Assessment Category	Potential Indicators of This Nutrition Diagnosis (one or more must be present)
Biochemical Data, Medical Tests and Procedures	• ↑ Triene:tetraene ratio > 0.2
Anthropometric Measurements	• Impaired growth • Weight loss if insufficient calories/kcal/kJ consumed
Nutrition-Focused Physical Findings	• Scaly skin and dermatitis consistent with essential fatty acid deficiency

Arrows used with laboratory values: ↑ represents above reference standard and ↓ represents below reference standard.

If a synonym for the term "inadequate" is helpful or needed, an approved alternate is the word "suboptimal."

DIAGNOSIS

Inadequate* Fat Intake (NI-5.6.1)

Food/Nutrition-Related History	Reports or observations of: • Estimated intake of essential fatty acids less than 10% of energy (primarily associated with parenteral nutrition) • Verbalizes inaccurate or incomplete knowledge • Cultural or religious practices that affect intake
Client History	• Conditions associated with a diagnosis or treatment, e.g., prolonged catabolic illness (e.g., AIDS, tuberculosis, anorexia nervosa, sepsis or severe infection from recent surgery) • Severe fat malabsorption with bowel resection, pancreatic insufficiency, or hepatic disease accompanied by steatorrhea

Updated: 2013 Edition

DIAGNOSIS

*If a synonym for the term "inadequate" is helpful or needed, an approved alternate is the word "suboptimal."

Excessive Fat Intake (NI-5.6.2)

Definition

Higher fat intake compared to established reference standards or recommendations based on physiological needs.

Etiology (Cause/Contributing Risk Factors)

Factors gathered during the nutrition assessment process that contribute to the existence or the maintenance of pathophysiological, psychosocial, situational, developmental, cultural, and/or environmental problems:

- Food- and nutrition-related knowledge deficit concerning appropriate amount of dietary fat
- Unsupported beliefs/attitudes about food, nutrition, and nutrition-related topics
- Lack of or limited access to healthful food choices, e.g., healthful food choices not provided as an option by caregiver or parent, homeless
- Changes in taste and appetite or preference
- Lack of value for behavior change, competing values
- Physiological causes decreasing total fat needs or recommendations

Signs/Symptoms (Defining Characteristics)

A typical cluster of subjective and objective signs and symptoms gathered during the nutrition assessment process that provide evidence that a problem exists; quantify the problem and describe its severity.

Nutrition Assessment Category	Potential Indicators of This Nutrition Diagnosis (one or more must be present)
Biochemical Data, Medical Tests and Procedures	• ↑ Cholesterol > 200 mg/dL (5.2 mmol/L), ↑ LDL cholesterol > 100 mg/dL (2.59 mmol/L), ↓ HDL cholesterol < 40 mg/dL (1.036 mmol/L), ↑ triglycerides > 150 mg/dL (1.695 mmol/L) • ↑ Serum amylase and/or lipase • ↑ LFTs, T. bilirubin • ↑ Fecal fat > 7g/24 hours
Anthropometric Measurements	
Nutrition-Focused Physical Findings	• Evidence of xanthomas • Diarrhea, cramping, steatorrhea, epigastric pain

Arrows used with laboratory values: ↑ represents above reference standard and ↓ represents below reference standard.

Excessive Fat Intake (NI-5.6.2)

Food/Nutrition-Related History	Reports or observations of: • Frequent or large portions of high-fat foods • Frequent food preparation with added fat • Frequent consumption of high-risk lipids (i.e., saturated fat, *trans* fat, cholesterol) • Report of foods containing fat more than diet prescription • Medication, e.g., pancreatic enzymes, cholesterol- or other lipid-lowering medications • Verbalizes inaccurate or incomplete knowledge • Verbalizes unsupported beliefs and attitudes
Client History	• Conditions associated with a diagnosis or treatment, e.g., hyperlipidemia; cystic fibrosis; angina; atherosclerosis; pancreatic; liver; and biliary diseases; post-transplantation, chyle fluid leak • Family history of hyperlipidemia, atherosclerosis, or pancreatitis

DIAGNOSIS

Updated: 2013 Edition

Less than Optimal Intake of Types of Fats (Specify) (NI-5.6.3)

Definition

Intake of wrong type or quality of fats compared to established reference standards or recommendations based on physiological needs.

Etiology (Cause/Contributing Risk Factors)

Factors gathered during the nutrition assessment process that contribute to the existence or the maintenance of pathophysiological, psychosocial, situational, developmental, cultural, and/or environmental problems:

- Food- and nutrition-related knowledge deficit concerning type of fat (e.g., fats added to food, formula/breastmilk)
- Unsupported beliefs/attitudes about food, nutrition, and nutrition-related topics
- Lack of or limited access to healthful food choices, e.g., healthful food choices not provided as an option by caregiver or parent, homeless
- Changes in taste and appetite or preference
- Lack of value for behavior change, competing values
- Physiological causes altering fatty acid needs or recommendations

Signs/Symptoms (Defining Characteristics)

A typical cluster of subjective and objective signs and symptoms gathered during the nutrition assessment process that provide evidence that a problem exists; quantify the problem and describe its severity.

Nutrition Assessment Category	Potential Indicators of This Nutrition Diagnosis (one or more must be present)
Biochemical Data, Medical Tests and Procedures	• ↑ Cholesterol > 200 mg/dL (5.2 mmol/L), ↑ LDL cholesterol > 100 mg/dL (2.59 mmol/L), ↓ HDL cholesterol < 40 mg/dL (1.036 mmol/L) men, ↓ HDL cholesterol < 50 mg/dL (1.3 mmol/L) women, ↑ triglycerides > 150 mg/dL (1.695 mmol/L) • ↑ Serum amylase and/or lipase • ↑ LFTs, T. bilirubin, C-reactive protein
Anthropometric Measurements	
Nutrition-Focused Physical Findings	• Evidence of dermatitis • Diarrhea, cramping, steatorrhea, epigastric pain

Arrows used with laboratory values: ↑ represents above reference standard and ↓ represents below reference standard

Less than Optimal Intake of Types of Fats (Specify) (NI-5.6.3)

Food/Nutrition-Related History	Reports or observations of: • Frequent food preparation with added fat that is not of desired type for condition • Frequent consumption of fats that are undesirable for condition (e.g., saturated fat, *trans* fat, cholesterol, n-6 fatty acids, long-chain fatty acids) • Estimated intake of monounsaturated, polyunsaturated, n-3 fatty acids, or DHA/ARA less than recommended or in suboptimal ratio • Verbalizes inaccurate or incomplete knowledge • Verbalizes unsupported beliefs and attitudes
Client History	• Conditions associated with a diagnosis or treatment, e.g., diabetes, cardiac diseases, obesity, liver or biliary disorders, chyle fluid leak • Family history of diabetes-related heart disease, hyperlipidemia, atherosclerosis, or pancreatitis

DIAGNOSIS

Updated: 2013 Edition

Inadequate* Protein Intake (NI-5.7.1)

Definition
Lower intake of protein compared to established reference standards or recommendations based on physiological needs.

> *Note: Whenever possible, nutrient intake data should be considered in combination with clinical, biochemical, anthropometric information, medical diagnosis, clinical status, and/or other factors as well as diet to provide a valid assessment of nutritional status based on a totality of the evidence. (Institute of Medicine. Dietary Reference Intakes: Applications in Dietary Assessment. Washington, DC: National Academies Press; 2000.)*

Etiology (Cause/Contributing Risk Factors)
Factors gathered during the nutrition assessment process that contribute to the existence or the maintenance of pathophysiological, psychosocial, situational, developmental, cultural, and/or environmental problems:

- Physiological causes increasing nutrient needs due to prolonged catabolic illness, malabsorption, age, or condition
- Decreased ability to consume sufficient protein
- Lack of or limited access to food, e.g., economic constraints, restricting food given to elderly and/or children
- Cultural practices that affect the ability to access food
- Food- and nutrition-related knowledge deficit concerning amount of protein
- Psychological causes such as depression and disordered eating

Signs/Symptoms (Defining Characteristics)
A typical cluster of subjective and objective signs and symptoms gathered during the nutrition assessment process that provide evidence that a problem exists; quantify the problem and describe its severity.

Nutrition Assessment Category	Potential Indicators of This Nutrition Diagnosis (one or more must be present)
Biochemical Data, Medical Tests and Procedures	
Anthropometric Measurements	
Nutrition-Focused Physical Findings	• Edema, failure to thrive (infants/children), poor musculature, dull skin, thin and fragile hair

*If a synonym for the term "inadequate" is helpful or needed, an approved alternate is the word "suboptimal."

Inadequate* Protein Intake (NI-5.7.1)

Food/Nutrition-Related History	Reports or observation of: • Estimated intake of protein insufficient to meet requirements • Cultural or religious practices that limit protein intake • Economic constraints that limit food availability • Prolonged adherence to a very low-protein weight-loss diet • Verbalizes inaccurate or incomplete knowledge
Client History	• Conditions associated with a diagnosis or treatment, e.g., severe protein malabsorption such as bowel resection

Updated: 2011 Edition

DIAGNOSIS

*If a synonym for the term "inadequate" is helpful or needed, an approved alternate is the word "suboptimal."

4th Edition

Excessive Protein Intake (NI-5.7.2)

Definition
Intake more than the recommended level of protein compared to established reference standards or recommendations based on physiological needs.

Etiology (Cause/Contributing Risk Factors)
Factors gathered during the nutrition assessment process that contribute to the existence or the maintenance of pathophysiological, psychosocial, situational, developmental, cultural, and/or environmental problems:

- Liver dysfunction
- Renal dysfunction
- Unsupported beliefs/attitudes about food, nutrition, and nutrition-related topics
- Food and nutrition-related knowledge deficit
- Lack of, or limited access to specialized protein products
- Metabolic abnormality
- Food faddism

Signs/Symptoms (Defining Characteristics)
A typical cluster of subjective and objective signs and symptoms gathered during the nutrition assessment process that provide evidence that a problem exists; quantify the problem and describe its severity.

Nutrition Assessment Category	Potential Indicators of This Nutrition Diagnosis (one or more must be present)
Biochemical Data, Medical Tests and Procedures	• Altered laboratory values, e.g., ↑ BUN, ↓ glomerular filtration rate (altered renal status)
Anthropometric Measurements	• Growth stunting or failure based on National Center for Health Statistics growth charts (metabolic disorders)
Nutrition-Focused Physical Findings	
Food/Nutrition-Related History	Reports or observations of: • Estimated total protein intake higher than recommended, e.g., early renal disease, advanced liver disease with confusion • Less than optimal supplementation • Verbalizes inaccurate or incomplete knowledge • Verbalizes unsupported beliefs and attitudes
Client History	• Conditions associated with a diagnosis or treatment, e.g., early renal disease or advanced liver disease with confusion

Arrows used with laboratory values: ↑ represents above reference standard and ↓ represents below reference standard.

Updated: 2013 Edition

Less than Optimal Intake of Types of Proteins or Amino Acids (Specify) (NI-5.7.3)

Definition

Intake of an amount of a specific type of protein or amino acid compared to established reference standards or recommendations based on physiological needs.

Etiology (Cause/Contributing Risk Factors)

Factors gathered during the nutrition assessment process that contribute to the existence or the maintenance of pathophysiological, psychosocial, situational, developmental, cultural, and/or environmental problems:

- Liver dysfunction
- Renal dysfunction
- Unsupported beliefs/attitudes about food, nutrition, and nutrition-related topics
- Misused specialized protein products
- Metabolic abnormality
- Food faddism
- Inborn errors of metabolism
- Celiac disease, dermatitis herpetiformis
- Cultural or religious practices that affect the ability to regulate types of protein or amino acids consumed
- Food- and nutrition-related knowledge deficit concerning an appropriate amount of a specific types of proteins or amino acids
- Food and nutrition compliance limitations, e.g., lack of willingness or failure to modify protein or amino acid intake in response to recommendations from a dietitian, physician, or caregiver

Signs/Symptoms (Defining Characteristics)

A typical cluster of subjective and objective signs and symptoms gathered during the nutrition assessment process that provide evidence that a problem exists; quantify the problem and describe its severity.

Nutrition Assessment Category	Potential Indicators of This Nutrition Diagnosis (one or more must be present)
Biochemical Data, Medical Tests and Procedures	Altered laboratory values, e.g., ↑ BUN, ↓ glomerular filtration rate (altered renal status) • ↑ specific amino acids (inborn errors of metabolism) • ↑ homocysteine or ammonia • Positive autoantibody levels (Anti-tTG antibodies, EmA IgA tissue transglutaminase [tTG] and IgA endomysial antibodies [EMA]) • Positive small bowel biopsy for celiac disease

Arrows used with laboratory values: ↑ *represents above reference standard and* ↓ *represents below reference standard.*

Less than Optimal Intake of Types of Proteins or Amino Acids (Specify) (NI-5.7.3)

Anthropometric Measurements	• Weight loss, inability to gain weight, delayed growth
Nutrition-Focused Physical Findings	• Physical or neurological changes (inborn errors of metabolism) • Diarrhea in response to certain types of carbohydrates • Abdominal pain, distention, constipation, reflux, GERD
Food/Nutrition-Related History	Reports or observation of: • Estimated protein or amino acid intake higher than recommended, e.g., early renal disease, advanced liver disease, inborn error of metabolism, celiac disease, food allergy or intolerance • Estimated intake of certain types of proteins or amino acids higher than recommended for prescribed parenteral and enteral nutrition therapy • Less than optimal amino acid or protein supplementation, as for athletes • Estimated amino acid intake higher than recommended, e.g., excess phenylalanine intake • Limited knowledge of protein or amino acid composition of foods or of protein or amino acid metabolism • Chronic use of medications containing proteins not recommended
Client History	• Conditions associated with a diagnosis or treatment of illness that requires EN/PN therapy, celiac disease, dermatitis herpetiformis, allergies, inborn errors of metabolism • History of inborn error of metabolism • Uremia, azotemia (renal patients)

Updated: 2013 Edition

Inadequate* Carbohydrate Intake (NI-5.8.1)

Definition

Lower intake of carbohydrate compared to established reference standards or recommendations based on physiological needs.

> Note: Whenever possible, nutrient intake data should be considered in combination with clinical, biochemical, anthropometric information, medical diagnosis, clinical status, and/or other factors as well as diet to provide a valid assessment of nutritional status based on a totality of the evidence. (Institute of Medicine. Dietary Reference Intakes: Applications in Dietary Assessment. *Washington, DC: National Academies Press; 2000.*)

Etiology (Cause/Contributing Risk Factors)

Factors gathered during the nutrition assessment process that contribute to the existence or the maintenance of pathophysiological, psychosocial, situational, developmental, cultural, and/or environmental problems:

- Physiological causes, e.g., increased energy needs due to increased activity level or metabolic change, malabsorption
- Lack of or limited access to food, e.g., economic constraints, restricting food given to elderly and/or children
- Cultural practices that affect the ability to access food
- Food- and nutrition-related knowledge deficit concerning appropriate amount of dietary carbohydrate
- Psychological causes such as depression and disordered eating

Signs/Symptoms (Defining Characteristics)

A typical cluster of subjective and objective signs and symptoms gathered during the nutrition assessment process that provide evidence that a problem exists; quantify the problem and describe its severity.

Nutrition Assessment Category	Potential Indicators of This Nutrition Diagnosis (one or more must be present)
Biochemical Data, Medical Tests and Procedures	
Anthropometric Measurements	
Nutrition-Focused Physical Findings	• Ketone smell on breath

*If a synonym for the term "inadequate" is helpful or needed, an approved alternate is the word "suboptimal."

Inadequate* Carbohydrate Intake (NI-5.8.1)

Food/Nutrition-Related History	Reports or observation of: • Estimated carbohydrate intake less than recommended amounts • Inability to independently consume foods/fluids, e.g., diminished mobility in hand, wrist, or digits • Verbalizes inaccurate or incomplete knowledge
Client History	• Conditions associated with a diagnosis or treatment, e.g., pancreatic insufficiency, hepatic disease, celiac disease, seizure disorder, or carbohydrate malabsorption

Updated: 2013 Edition

If a synonym for the term "inadequate" is helpful or needed, an approved alternate is the word "suboptimal."

Excessive Carbohydrate Intake (NI-5.8.2)

Definition

Intake more than the recommended level and type of carbohydrate compared to established reference standards or recommendations based on physiological needs.

Etiology (Cause/Contributing Risk Factors)

Factors gathered during the nutrition assessment process that contribute to the existence or the maintenance of pathophysiological, psychosocial, situational, developmental, cultural, and/or environmental problems:

- Physiological causes requiring modified carbohydrate intake, e.g., diabetes mellitus, lactase deficiency, sucrase-isomaltase deficiency, aldolase-B deficiency
- Cultural practices that affect the ability to reduce carbohydrate intake
- Food- and nutrition-related knowledge deficit concerning appropriate amount of carbohydrate intake
- Food and nutrition compliance limitations, e.g., lack of willingness or failure to modify carbohydrate intake in response to recommendations from a dietitian or physician
- Psychological causes such as depression and disordered eating

Signs/Symptoms (Defining Characteristics)

A typical cluster of subjective and objective signs and symptoms gathered during the nutrition assessment process that provide evidence that a problem exists; quantify the problem and describe its severity.

Nutrition Assessment Category	Potential Indicators of This Nutrition Diagnosis (one or more must be present)
Biochemical Data, Medical Tests and Procedures	• Hyperglycemia ($\uparrow$ fasting blood glucose > 126 mg/dL) • $\uparrow$ Hemoglobin A1C > 6% • $\uparrow$ Oral glucose tolerance test (2-hour post load glucose > 200 mg/dL)
Anthropometric Measurements	
Nutrition-Focused Physical Findings	• Dental caries • Diarrhea in response to carbohydrate feeding

Arrows used with laboratory values: $\uparrow$ represents above reference standard and $\downarrow$ represents below reference standard.

4th Edition

Excessive Carbohydrate Intake (NI-5.8.2)

Food/Nutrition-Related History	Reports or observation of: • Cultural or religious practices that do not support modification of dietary carbohydrate intake • Estimated carbohydrate intake that is consistently more than recommended amounts • Chronic use of medications that cause hyperglycemia, e.g., steroids • Verbalizes inaccurate or incomplete knowledge
Client History	• Conditions associated with a diagnosis or treatment, e.g., diabetes mellitus, inborn errors of carbohydrate metabolism, lactase deficiency, severe infection, sepsis, or obesity • Pancreatic insufficiency resulting in reduced insulin production • Economic constraints that limit availability of appropriate foods

Updated: 2013 Edition

DIAGNOSIS

Less than Optimal Intake of Types of Carbohydrates (Specify) (NI-5.8.3)

Definition
Intake of an amount of a specific type of carbohydrate compared to the established reference standards or recommendations based on physiological needs.

> *Note: Types of carbohydrate can refer generally to sugars, starch and fiber or specific carbohydrates (e.g., sucrose, fructose, lactose). Intolerance to the protein component of grains (e.g., gluten) should be documented using the Less than optimal intake of types of proteins or amino acids (NI-5.7.3) reference sheet.*

Etiology (Cause/Contributing Risk Factors)
Factors gathered during the nutrition assessment process that contribute to the existence or the maintenance of pathophysiological, psychosocial, situational, developmental, cultural, and/or environmental problems:

- Physiological causes requiring careful use of modified carbohydrate, e.g., intolerance, inborn errors of carbohydrate metabolism.
  > *Note. Although research does not support restriction of individual types of carbohydrate for glycemic control, food and nutrition professionals may determine that restriction is warranted in unique patient/client situations for glycemic control and/ or for other reasons, such as promotion of healthful eating.*

- Cultural or religious practices that affect the ability to regulate types of carbohydrate consumed

- Food- and nutrition-related knowledge deficit concerning an appropriate amount of a specific type of carbohydrate

- Food and nutrition compliance limitations, e.g., lack of willingness or failure to modify carbohydrate intake in response to recommendations from a dietitian, physician, or caregiver

- Psychological causes such as depression and disordered eating

Signs/Symptoms (Defining Characteristics)
A typical cluster of subjective and objective signs and symptoms gathered during the nutrition assessment process that provide evidence that a problem exists; quantify the problem and describe its severity.

Nutrition Assessment Category	Potential Indicators of This Nutrition Diagnosis (one or more must be present)
Biochemical Data, Medical Tests and Procedures	• Hypoglycemia or hyperglycemia
Anthropometric Measurements	• Weight loss, inability to gain weight, delayed growth
Nutrition-Focused Physical Findings	• Diarrhea in response to certain types of carbohydrates • Abdominal pain, distention, constipation, reflux, GERD

DIAGNOSIS

Less than Optimal Intake of Types of Carbohydrates (Specify) (NI-5.8.3)

Food/Nutrition-Related History	Reports or observations of: • Carbohydrate intake that is a different type or exceeds amount recommended for that specific type of carbohydrate • Limited knowledge of carbohydrate composition of foods or of carbohydrate metabolism • Chronic use of medications that cause altered glucose levels, e.g., steroids, antidepressants, antipsychotics, or contains a type of carbohydrate not recommended • Cultural or religious practices that affect intake
Client History	• Conditions associated with a diagnosis or treatment, e.g., intolerance, inborn errors of metabolism • Allergic reactions or intolerance to certain carbohydrate foods or food groups • Economic constraints that limit availability of appropriate foods

Updated: 2013 Edition

Inconsistent Carbohydrate Intake (NI-5.8.4)

Definition

Inconsistent timing of carbohydrate intake throughout the day, day to day, or a pattern of carbohydrate intake that is not consistent with recommended pattern based on physiological or medication needs.

Etiology (Cause/Contributing Risk Factors)

Factors gathered during the nutrition assessment process that contribute to the existence or the maintenance of pathophysiological, psychosocial, situational, developmental, cultural, and/or environmental problems:

- Physiological causes requiring careful timing and consistency in the amount of carbohydrate, e.g., diabetes mellitus, hypoglycemia, PN/EN delivery
- Cultural practices that affect the ability to regulate timing of carbohydrate consumption
- Food- and nutrition-related knowledge deficit concerning appropriate timing of carbohydrate intake
- Food and nutrition compliance limitations, e.g., lack of willingness or failure to modify carbohydrate timing in response to recommendations from a dietitian, physician, or caregiver
- Psychological causes such as depression and disordered eating

Signs/Symptoms (Defining Characteristics)

A typical cluster of subjective and objective signs and symptoms gathered during the nutrition assessment process that provide evidence that a problem exists; quantify the problem and describe its severity.

Nutrition Assessment Category	Potential Indicators of This Nutrition Diagnosis (one or more must be present)
Biochemical Data, Medical Tests and Procedures	• Hypoglycemia or hyperglycemia documented on regular basis associated with inconsistent carbohydrate intake • Wide variations in blood glucose levels
Anthropometric Measurements	
Nutrition-Focused Physical Findings	

DIAGNOSIS

Inconsistent Carbohydrate Intake (NI-5.8.4)

Food/Nutrition-Related History	Reports or observations of: • Estimated carbohydrate intake that is different from recommended types or ingested on an irregular basis • Use of insulin or insulin secretagogues • Chronic use of medications that cause altered glucose levels, e.g., steroids, antidepressants, antipsychotics • Verbalizes inaccurate or incomplete knowledge • Cultural or religious practices that affect intake
Client History	• Conditions associated with a diagnosis or treatment, e.g., diabetes mellitus, obesity, metabolic syndrome, hypoglycemia • Economic constraints that limit availability of appropriate foods

Updated: 2013 Edition

Inadequate* Fiber Intake (NI-5.8.5)

Definition

Lower intake of fiber compared to established reference standards or recommendations based on physiological needs.

> Note: Whenever possible, nutrient intake data should be considered in combination with clinical, biochemical, anthropometric information, medical diagnosis, clinical status, and/or other factors as well as diet to provide a valid assessment of nutritional status based on a totality of the evidence. (Institute of Medicine. Dietary Reference Intakes: Applications in Dietary Assessment. Washington, DC: National Academies Press; 2000.)

Etiology (Cause/Contributing Risk Factors)

Factors gathered during the nutrition assessment process that contribute to the existence or the maintenance of pathophysiological, psychosocial, situational, developmental, cultural, and/or environmental problems:

- Lack of or limited access to fiber-containing foods/fluids
- Food- and nutrition-related knowledge deficit concerning desirable quantities of fiber
- Psychological causes such as depression and disordered eating
- Prolonged adherence to a low-fiber or low-residue diet
- Difficulty chewing or swallowing high-fiber foods
- Economic constraints that limit availability of appropriate foods
- Inability or unwillingness to purchase or consume fiber-containing foods
- Less than optimal food-preparation practices, e.g., reliance on overprocessed, overcooked foods

Signs/Symptoms (Defining Characteristics)

A typical cluster of subjective and objective signs and symptoms gathered during the nutrition assessment process that provide evidence that a problem exists; quantify the problem and describe its severity.

Nutrition Assessment Category	Potential Indicators of This Nutrition Diagnosis (one or more must be present)
Biochemical Data, Medical Tests and Procedures	
Anthropometric Measurements	
Nutrition-Focused Physical Findings	• Inadequate fecal bulk

*If a synonym for the term "inadequate" is helpful or needed, an approved alternate is the word "suboptimal."

4th Edition

DIAGNOSIS

Inadequate* Fiber Intake (NI-5.8.5)

Food/Nutrition-Related History	Reports or observations of: • Estimated intake of fiber that is insufficient when compared to recommended amounts (38 g/day for men and 25 g/day for women) • Verbalizes inaccurate or incomplete knowledge
Client History	• Conditions associated with a diagnosis or treatment, e.g., ulcer disease, inflammatory bowel disease, or short-bowel syndrome treated with a low-fiber diet

Updated: 2013 Edition

If a synonym for the term "inadequate" is helpful or needed, an approved alternate is the word "suboptimal."

Excessive Fiber Intake (NI-5.8.6)

Definition

Higher intake of fiber compared to recommendations based on patient/client condition.

Etiology (Cause/Contributing Risk Factors)

Factors gathered during the nutrition assessment process that contribute to the existence or the maintenance of pathophysiological, psychosocial, situational, developmental, cultural, and/or environmental problems:

- Food- and nutrition-related knowledge deficit concerning desirable quantities of fiber
- Unsupported beliefs or attitudes about food- or nutrition-related topics, e.g., obsession with bowel frequency and habits
- Lack of knowledge about appropriate fiber intake for condition
- Food preparation or eating patterns that involve only high-fiber foods to the exclusion of other nutrient-dense foods

Signs/Symptoms (Defining Characteristics)

A typical cluster of subjective and objective signs and symptoms gathered during the nutrition assessment process that provide evidence that a problem exists; quantify the problem and describe its severity.

Nutrition Assessment Category	Potential Indicators of This Nutrition Diagnosis (one or more must be present)
Biochemical Data, Medical Tests and Procedures	
Anthropometric Measurements	
Nutrition-Focused Physical Findings	• Nausea, vomiting, excessive flatulence, diarrhea, abdominal cramping, high stool volume or frequency that causes discomfort to the individual
Food/Nutrition-Related History	Reports or observations of: • Estimated fiber intake higher than tolerated or generally recommended for current medical condition • Verbalizes inaccurate or incomplete knowledge • Verbalizes unsupported beliefs and attitudes
Client History	• Conditions associated with a diagnosis or treatment, e.g., ulcer disease, irritable bowel syndrome, inflammatory bowel disease, short-bowel syndrome, diverticulitis, obstructive constipation, prolapsing hemorrhoids, gastrointestinal stricture, eating disorders, or mental illness with obsessive-compulsive tendencies • Obstruction, phytobezoar

DIAGNOSIS

Updated: 2013 Edition

Inadequate* Vitamin Intake (Specify) (NI-5.9.1)

Definition

Lower intake of one or more vitamins compared to established reference standards or recommendations based on physiological needs.

> *Note: Whenever possible, nutrient intake data should be considered in combination with clinical, biochemical, anthropometric information, medical diagnosis, clinical status, and/or other factors as well as diet to provide a valid assessment of nutritional status based on a totality of the evidence. (Institute of Medicine.* Dietary Reference Intakes: Applications in Dietary Assessment. *Washington, DC: National Academies Press; 2000.)*

Etiology (Cause/Contributing Risk Factors)

Factors gathered during the nutrition assessment process that contribute to the existence or the maintenance of pathophysiological, psychosocial, situational, developmental, cultural, and/or environmental problems:

- Physiological causes increasing nutrient needs, e.g., due to prolonged catabolic illness, disease state, malabsorption, or medications
- Decreased ability to consume sufficient amount of a vitamin(s)
- Lack of or limited access to food, e.g., economic constraints, restricting food given to elderly and/or children
- Cultural practices that affect ability to access food
- Food- and nutrition-related knowledge deficit concerning food and supplemental sources of vitamins
- Psychological causes, e.g., depression or eating disorders
- Access causes including season, geography, limited access to sunlight

Signs/Symptoms (Defining Characteristics)

A typical cluster of subjective and objective signs and symptoms gathered during the nutrition assessment process that provide evidence that a problem exists; quantify the problem and describe its severity.

If a synonym for the term "inadequate" is helpful or needed, an approved alternate is the word "suboptimal."

Inadequate* Vitamin Intake (Specify) (NI-5.9.1)

Nutrition Assessment Category	Potential Indicators of This Nutrition Diagnosis (one or more must be present)
Biochemical Data, Medical Tests and Procedures	• Vitamin A: ↓ serum retinol < 10 µg/dL (0.35 µmol/L) • Vitamin C: ↓ plasma concentrations < 0.2 mg/dL (11.4 µmol/L) • Vitamin D: ↓ 25(OH)D <50 nmol/L, ↓ ionized calcium < 3.9 mg/dL (0.98 mmol/L) with ↑ parathyroid hormone, normal serum calcium, and ↓ serum phosphorus < 2.6 mg/dL (0.84 mmol/L) • Vitamin E: ↓ plasma alpha-tocopherol < 18 µmol/g (41.8 µmol/L) • Vitamin K: ↑ prothrombin time; altered INR (without anticoagulation therapy) • Thiamin: ↑ erythrocyte transketolase activity > 1.20 µg/mL/h • Riboflavin: ↑ erythrocyte glutathione reductase > 1.2 IU/g hemoglobin • Niacin: ↓ N'methyl-nicotinamide excretion < 5.8 µmol/day • Vitamin B-6: ↓ plasma pryrdoxal 5'phosphate <5 ng/mL (20 nmol/L) • Vitamin B-12: ↓ serum concentration < 24.4 ng/dL (180 pmol/L); ↑ homocysteine • Folic acid: ↓ serum concentration < 0.3 µg/dL (7 nmol/L); ↓ red cell folate < 315 nmol/L • Pantothenic acid: ↓ plasma • Biotin: ↓ serum
Anthropometric Measurements	
Nutrition-Focused Physical Findings	• Vitamin A: night blindness, Bitot's spots, xerophthalmia, follicular hyperkeratosis • Vitamin C: follicular hyperkeratosis, petichiae, ecchymosis, coiled hairs, inflamed and bleeding gums, perifolicular hemorrhages, joint effusions, arthralgia, and impaired wound healing • Vitamin D: widening at ends of long bones • Riboflavin: sore throat, hyperemia, edema of pharyngeal and oral mucous membranes, cheilosis, angular stomatitis, glossitis, magenta tongue, seborrheic dermatitis, and normochromic, normocytic anemia with pure erythrocyte cytoplasia of the bone marrow

DIAGNOSIS

Arrows used with laboratory values: ↑ *represents above reference standard and* ↓ *represents below reference standard.*

If a synonym for the term "inadequate" is helpful or needed, an approved alternate is the word "suboptimal."

4th Edition

Inadequate* Vitamin Intake (Specify) (NI-5.9.1)

Nutrition-Focused Physical Findings, cont'd	• Niacin: symmetrical, pigmented rash on areas exposed to sunlight; bright red tongue • Vitamin B-6: seborrheic dermatitis, stomatitis, cheilosis, glossitis, confusion, depression • Vitamin B-12: tingling and numbness in extremities, diminished vibratory and position sense, motor disturbances including gait disturbances • Pantothenic acid: irritability and restlessness, fatigue, apathy, malaise, sleep disturbances, nausea, vomiting, abdominal cramps, numbness, muscle cramps, hypoglycemia, sensitivity to insulin • Biotin: dermatitis, conjunctivitis, alopecia, depression, lethargy, hallucinations and paresthesia, hypotonia, developmental delays
Food/Nutrition-Related History	Reports or observations of: • Estimated intake of foods containing specific vitamins less than requirements or recommended level • Intake of foods that do not contain available vitamins, e.g., over processed, overcooked, or improperly stored foods • Prolonged use of substances known to increase vitamin requirements or reduce vitamin absorption • Lack of interest in foods
Client History	• Conditions associated with a diagnosis or treatment, e.g., malabsorption as a result of celiac disease, short-bowel syndrome, or inflammatory bowel • Certain environmental conditions, e.g., infants exclusively fed breastmilk with limited exposure to sunlight (Vitamin D) • History of chronic kidney disease (decreased conversion of 25(OH)D • Premature infant, extremely low-birth-weight infant (vitamin D) • Rachitic rosary in children, rickets, osteomalacia • Pellegra • Vitamin/mineral deficiency

Updated: 2013 Edition

If a synonym for the term "inadequate" is helpful or needed, an approved alternate is the word "suboptimal."

Excessive Vitamin Intake (Specify) (NI-5.9.2)

Definition

Higher intake of one or more vitamins compared to established reference standards or recommendations based on physiological needs.

Etiology (Cause/Contributing Risk Factors)

Factors gathered during the nutrition assessment process that contribute to the existence or the maintenance of pathophysiological, psychosocial, situational, developmental, cultural, and/or environmental problems:

- Physiological causes decreasing nutrient needs due to prolonged immobility or chronic renal disease
- Access to foods and supplements in excess of needs, e.g., cultural or religious practices; less-than-optimal food and supplements given to pregnant women, elderly, or children
- Food- and nutrition-related knowledge deficit concerning food and supplemental sources of vitamins
- Psychological causes, e.g., depression or eating disorders
- Accidental overdose from oral and supplemental forms, enteral or parenteral sources

Signs/Symptoms (Defining Characteristics)

A typical cluster of subjective and objective signs and symptoms gathered during the nutrition assessment process that provide evidence that a problem exists; quantify the problem and describe its severity.

Nutrition Assessment Category	Potential Indicators of This Nutrition Diagnosis (one or more must be present)
Biochemical Data, Medical Tests and Procedures	• Vitamin D: ↑ 25(OH) D, ↑ ionized calcium > 5.4 mg/dL (1.35 mmol/L) with ↑ parathyroid hormone, normal or ↑ serum calcium, and ↑ serum phosphorus > 2.6 mg/dL (0.84 mmol/L) • Vitamin K: ↓ prothrombin time or altered INR • Niacin: ↑ N'methyl-nicotinamide excretion > 7.3 μmol/day • Vitamin B-6: ↑ plasma pryrdoxal 5'phosphate > 15.7 ng/mL (94 nmol/L) • Vitamin A: ↑ serum retinol concentration > 60 μg/dL (2.09 μmol/L) • Pantothenic acid: ↑ plasma • Biotin: ↑ serum
Anthropometric Measurements	• Vitamin D: growth retardation

Arrows used with laboratory values: ↑ represents above reference standard and ↓ represents below reference standard.

Excessive Vitamin Intake (Specify) (NI-5.9.2)

Nutrition-Focused Physical Findings	• Vitamin A: changes in the skin and mucous membranes; dry lips (cheilitis); early—dryness of the nasal mucosa and eyes; later—dryness, erythema, scaling and peeling of the skin, hair loss, and nail fragility. Headache, nausea, and vomiting. Infants may have bulging fontanelle; children may develop bone alterations. • Vitamin D: calcification of soft tissues (calcinosis), including the kidney, lungs, heart, and even the tympanic membrane of the ear, which can result in deafness. Headache and nausea. Infants given excessive amounts of vitamin D may have gastrointestinal upset, bone fragility. • Vitamin K: hemolytic anemia in adults or severe jaundice in infants have been noted on rare occasions • Niacin: histamine release, which causes flushing, aggravation of asthma, or liver disease
Food/Nutrition-Related History	Reports or observations of: • Estimated intake reflects excessive intake of foods and supplements containing vitamins as compared to estimated requirements, including fortified cereals, meal replacements, vitamin-mineral supplements, other dietary supplements (e.g., fish liver oils or capsules), tube feeding, and/or parenteral solutions • Estimated intake > more than Tolerable Upper Limit (UL) for vitamin A based upon reference intake standard • Estimated intake more than UL for vitamin D based upon reference intake standard • Estimated intake more than UL for niacin based upon reference intake standard
Client History	• Conditions associated with a diagnosis or treatment, e.g., chronic liver or kidney diseases, heart failure, cancer

Updated: 2013 Edition

DIAGNOSIS

Inadequate* Mineral Intake (Specify) (NI-5.10.1)

Definition
Lower intake of one or more minerals compared to established reference standards or recommendations based on physiological needs.

> Note: Whenever possible, nutrient intake data should be considered in combination with clinical, biochemical, anthropometric information, medical diagnosis, clinical status, and/or other factors as well as diet to provide a valid assessment of nutritional status based on a totality of the evidence. (Institute of Medicine. Dietary Reference Intakes: Applications in Dietary Assessment. Washington, DC: National Academies Press; 2000.)

Etiology (Cause/Contributing Risk Factors)
Factors gathered during the nutrition assessment process that contribute to the existence or the maintenance of pathophysiological, psychosocial, situational, developmental, cultural, and/or environmental problems:

- Physiological causes increasing nutrient needs due to prolonged catabolic illness, malabsorption, hyperexcretion, nutrient/drug and nutrient/nutrient interaction, growth and maturation
- Decreased ability to consume sufficient amount of a mineral(s)
- Lack of or limited access to food, e.g., economic constraints, restricting food given to elderly and/or children
- Cultural practices that affect ability to access food
- Food- and nutrition-related knowledge deficit concerning food and supplemental sources of minerals
- Misdiagnosis of lactose intolerance/lactase deficiency; perception of conflicting nutrition messages; less than optimal reliance on supplements
- Psychological causes, e.g., depression or eating disorders
- Environmental causes, e.g., inadequately tested nutrient bioavailability of fortified foods, beverages, and supplements; less than optimal marketing of fortified foods/beverages/supplements as a substitute for natural food source of nutrient(s)

Signs/Symptoms (Defining Characteristics)
A typical cluster of subjective and objective signs and symptoms gathered during the nutrition assessment process that provide evidence that a problem exists; quantify the problem and describe its severity.

If a synonym for the term "inadequate" is helpful or needed, an approved alternate is the word "suboptimal."

DIAGNOSIS

Inadequate* Mineral Intake
(Specify) (NI-5.10.1)

Nutrition Assessment Category	Potential Indicators of This Nutrition Diagnosis (one or more must be present)
Biochemical Data, Medical Tests and Procedures	• Calcium: bone mineral content (BMC) ↓ the young adult mean. Hypocalciuria, serum 25(OH)D < 32 ng/mL • ↓ Phosphorus, < 2.6 mg/dL (0.84 mmol/L) • ↓ Ferritin in patient/client with a ↓ Mean Corpuscular Volume (MCV) • ↓ Zinc, plasma • ↓ Magnesium, <1.8 mg/dL (0.7 mmol/L) • Iron: ↓ hemoglobin < 13 g/L (2 mmol/L) (males); < 12 g/L (1.86 mmol/L) (females) • Iodine: ↓ urinary excretion < 100 µg/L (788 nmol/L) • Copper, : ↓ serum copper < 64 µg/dL (10 µmol/L) • ↓ Selenium, plasma • ↓ Fluoride, plasma • ↓ Manganese, serum • ↓ Molybdenum, serum • ↓ Boron, serum or plasma
Anthropometric Measurements	• Calcium: height loss • Iodine: growth abnormalities • Chromium: unintentional weight loss
Nutrition-Focused Physical Findings	• Calcium: hypertension, acute – hyperactive reflexes, tetany, muscle spasm, irregular heart rhythm • Iron :pallor of face, mucosa, pale gums, tachycardia, fatigue • Potassium – weakness, constipation, hypoactive reflexes • Phosphorous: fatigue, myalgia, ataxia, confusion, parasthesias • Zinc: dysgeusia, poor wound healing, skin lesions (buttocks, perianal area, mouth, nose, eyes), alopecia • Copper: depigmentation of hair and skin, osteoporosis • Selenium:depigmentation of hair and skin • Iodine: enlarged thyroid • Fluoride: dental caries • Manganese: dermatitis

Arrows used with laboratory values: ↑ *represents above reference standard and* ↓ *represents below reference standard*

*If a synonym for the term "inadequate" is helpful or needed, an approved alternate is the word "suboptimal."

Inadequate* Mineral Intake (Specify) (NI-5.10.1)

Food/Nutrition-Related History	Reports or observations of: • Estimated mineral intake from diet less than recommended intake • Food avoidance and/or elimination of whole food group(s) from diet • Lack of interest in food • Less than optimal food choices and/or chronic dieting behavior • Verbalizes inaccurate or incomplete knowledge • Cultural or religious practices that affect intake
Client History	• Conditions associated with a diagnosis or treatment, e.g., malabsorption as a result of celiac disease, short bowel syndrome, inflammatory bowel disease, or post-menopausal women without estrogen supplementation and increased calcium need, bariatric surgery, parenteral nutrition • Polycystic ovary syndrome, premenstrual syndrome, kidney stones, colon polyps • Other significant medical diagnoses and therapies • Geographic latitude and history of Ultraviolet-B exposure/use of sunscreen • Change in living environment/independence • Calcium: obesity • Vitamin/mineral deficiency

Updated: 2013 Edition

DIAGNOSIS

If a synonym for the term "inadequate" is helpful or needed, an approved alternate is the word "suboptimal."

4th Edition

Excessive Mineral Intake (Specify) (NI-5.10.2)

Definition
Higher intake of one or more minerals compared to established reference standards or recommendations based on physiological needs.

Etiology (Cause/Contributing Risk Factors)
Factors gathered during the nutrition assessment process that contribute to the existence or the maintenance of pathophysiological, psychosocial, situational, developmental, cultural, and/or environmental problems:

- Food- and nutrition-related knowledge deficit concerning food and supplemental sources of minerals
- Unsupported beliefs/attitudes about food, nutrition, and nutrition-related topics
- Food faddism
- Accidental oversupplementation
- Overconsumption of a limited variety of foods
- Lack of knowledge about management of diagnosed genetic disorder altering mineral homeostasis [hemochromatosis (iron), Wilson's disease (copper)]
- Lack of knowledge about management of diagnosed disease state requiring mineral restriction [cholestatic liver disease (copper and manganese), renal insufficiency (phosphorus, magnesium, potassium)]

Signs/Symptoms (Defining Characteristics)
A typical cluster of subjective and objective signs and symptoms gathered during the nutrition assessment process that provide evidence that a problem exists; quantify the problem and describe its severity.

Nutrition Assessment Category	Potential Indicators of This Nutrition Diagnosis (one or more must be present)
Biochemical Data, Medical Tests and Procedures	Changes in appropriate laboratory values, such as: • ↑ TSH (iodine supplementation) • ↓ HDL (zinc supplementation) • ↑ Serum ferritin and transferrin saturation (iron overload) • Hyperphosphatemia • Hypermagnesemia • Copper deficiency anemia (zinc) • ↑ Fluoride, plasma • ↑ Selenium, serum • ↑ Manganese, serum • ↑ Molybdenum, serum • ↑ Boron, serum or plasma

Arrows used with laboratory values: ↑ represents above reference standard and ↓ represents below reference standard.

Excessive Mineral Intake (Specify) (NI-5.10.2)

Anthropometric Measurements	
Nutrition-Focused Physical Findings	• Hair and nail changes (selenium) • Anorexia (zinc supplementation) • GI disturbances (iron, magnesium, copper, zinc, selenium, sulfate, iodine) • Enamel or skeletal fluorosis (fluoride) • Central nervous system effects (manganese) • Verbalizes inaccurate or incomplete knowledge • Verbalizes unsupported beliefs and attitudes
Food/Nutrition-Related History	Reports or observations of: • Estimated intake containing high amounts of mineral compared to reference intake standard (e.g., DRIs)
Client History	• Liver damage (copper, iron) • Parenteral nutrition

Updated: 2013 Edition

DIAGNOSIS

Predicted Suboptimal Nutrient Intake (Specify) (NI-5.11.1)

Definition
Future intake of one or more nutrients that is anticipated, based on observation, experience, or scientific reason, to fall short of estimated nutrient requirements, established reference standards, or recommendations based on physiological needs.

Etiology (Cause/Contributing Risk Factors)
Factors gathered during the nutrition assessment process that contribute to the existence or the maintenance of pathophysiological, psychosocial, situational, developmental, cultural, and/or environmental problems:

- Scheduled or planned medical therapy or medication that is predicted to increase nutrient requirements
- Scheduled or planned medical therapy or medication that is predicted to decrease ability to consume sufficient nutrients
- Physiological condition associated with increased need for a nutrient due to altered metabolism
- Cultural or religious practices that will affect nutrient intake
- Anticipated isolated living/housing situation without routine access to a variety of nutritious foods
- Danger for environmental emergency or catastrophe/disaster

Signs/Symptoms (Defining Characteristics)
A typical cluster of subjective and objective signs and symptoms gathered during the nutrition assessment process that provide evidence that a problem exists; quantify the problem and describe its severity.

Nutrition Assessment Category	Potential Indicators of This Nutrition Diagnosis (one or more must be present)
Biochemical Data, Medical Tests and Procedures	• Population-based biochemical parameters indicating suboptimal nutrient intake
Anthropometric Measurements	• Population-based anthropometric data indicating suboptimal nutrient intake
Nutrition-Focused Physical Findings	• Population-based data on acute and chronic disease prevalence indicating suboptimal nutrient intake

Predicted Suboptimal Nutrient Intake (Specify) (NI-5.11.1)

Food/Nutrition-Related History	Reports or observations of: • Estimated nutrient(s) intake from all sources less than projected needs • History of marginal or suboptimal nutrient(s) intake • Projected change in ability to shop, prepare, and/or consume sufficient nutrient(s) • Medications that decrease appetite and/or affect ability to consume sufficient nutrient(s) • No prior knowledge of need for food- and nutrition-related recommendations • Religious or cultural practices that will affect nutrient intake • Low supplies in home in preparation for environmental emergency or catastrophe/disaster
Client History	• Scheduled surgical procedure or medical therapy known to increase nutrient(s) need or change ability to consume sufficient nutrient(s) • History or presence of a condition for which research shows an increased prevalence of insufficient nutrient(s) intake in a similar population • Isolated living/housing situation • Geographic location of home in location with danger for environmental emergency or catastrophe/disaster

Created: 2011 Edition

Predicted Excessive Nutrient Intake (Specify) (NI-5.11.2)

Definition

Future intake of one or more nutrients that is anticipated, based on observation, experience, or scientific reason, to be more than estimated nutrient requirements, established reference standards, or recommendations based on physiological needs.

Etiology (Cause/Contributing Risk Factors)

Factors gathered during the nutrition assessment process that contribute to the existence or the maintenance of pathophysiological, psychosocial, situational, developmental, cultural, and/or environmental problems:

- Scheduled or planned medical therapy or medication that is predicted to decrease nutrient requirements
- Anticipated physiological condition associated with reduced need for or altered metabolism of nutrients
- Scheduled or planned medical therapy or medication that is predicted to alter metabolism of nutrients

Signs/Symptoms (Defining Characteristics)

A typical cluster of subjective and objective signs and symptoms gathered during the nutrition assessment process that provide evidence that a problem exists; quantify the problem and describe its severity.

Nutrition Assessment Category	Potential Indicators of This Nutrition Diagnosis (one or more must be present)
Biochemical Data, Medical Tests and Procedures	• Population-based biochemical parameters indicating excessive nutrient intake
Anthropometric Measurements	• Population-based anthropometric data indicating excessive nutrient intake
Nutrition-Focused Physical Findings	• Population-based data on acute and chronic disease prevalence indicating excessive nutrient
Food/Nutrition-Related History	Reports or observations of: • Estimated nutrient(s) intake from all sources more than projected needs • History of excessive nutrient(s) intake • No prior knowledge of need for food- and nutrition-related recommendations

Predicted Excessive Nutrient Intake (Specify) (NI-5.11.2)

Client History	• Scheduled surgical procedure or medical therapy known to reduce nutrient(s) need or alter metabolism of a nutrient(s) • History or presence of a condition for which research shows an increased prevalence of excessive nutrient(s) intake in a similar population

Created: 2011 Edition

Swallowing Difficulty (NC-1.1)

Definition
Impaired or difficult movement of food and liquid within the oral cavity to the stomach

Etiology (Cause/Contributing Risk Factors)
Factors gathered during the nutrition assessment process that contribute to the existence or the maintenance of pathophysiological, psychosocial, situational, developmental, cultural, and/or environmental problems:

- Mechanical causes, e.g., inflammation, surgery, stricture; or oral, pharyngeal and esophageal tumors; prior mechanical ventilation
- Motor causes, e.g., neurological or muscular disorders, such as cerebral palsy, stroke, multiple sclerosis, scleroderma; or prematurity, altered suck, swallow, breathe patterns

Signs/Symptoms (Defining Characteristics)
A typical cluster of subjective and objective signs and symptoms gathered during the nutrition assessment process that provide evidence that a problem exists; quantify the problem and describe its severity.

Nutrition Assessment Category	Potential Indicators of This Nutrition Diagnosis (one or more must be present)
Biochemical Data, Medical Tests and Procedures	• Radiological findings, e.g., abnormal swallow study
Anthropometric Measurements	
Nutrition-Focused Physical Findings	• Evidence of dehydration, e.g., dry mucous membranes, poor skin turgor • Non-normal findings in cranial nerves and (CN VII) muscles of facial expression, (Nerve IX) gag reflex, swallow (Nerve X) and tongue range of motions (Nerve XII), cough reflex, drooling, facial weakness, and ability to perform and wet and dry swallow • Coughing, choking, prolonged chewing, pouching of food, regurgitation, facial expression changes during eating, drooling, noisy wet upper airway sounds, feeling of "food getting stuck," pain while swallowing
Food/Nutrition-Related History	Reports or observations of: • Prolonged feeding time • Decreased estimated food intake • Avoidance of foods • Mealtime resistance

DIAGNOSIS

Swallowing Difficulty (NC-1.1)

Client History	• Conditions associated with a diagnosis or treatment, e.g., dysphagia, achalasia • Repeated upper respiratory infections and or pneumonia

Updated: 2011 Edition

4th Edition

Biting/Chewing (Masticatory) Difficulty (NC-1.2)

Definition
Impaired ability to bite or chew food in preparation for swallowing.

Etiology (Cause/Contributing Risk Factors)
Factors gathered during the nutrition assessment process that contribute to the existence or the maintenance of pathophysiological, psychosocial, situational, developmental, cultural, and/or environmental problems:

- Craniofacial malformations
- Oral surgery
- Neuromuscular dysfunction
- Partial or complete edentulism
- Soft tissue disease (primary or oral manifestations of a systemic disease)
- Xerostomia

Signs/Symptoms (Defining Characteristics)
A typical cluster of subjective and objective signs and symptoms gathered during the nutrition assessment process that provide evidence that a problem exists; quantify the problem and describe its severity.

Nutrition Assessment Category	Potential Indicators of This Nutrition Diagnosis (one or more must be present)
Biochemical Data, Medical Tests and Procedures	
Anthropometric Measurements	
Nutrition-Focused Physical Findings	• Partial or complete edentulism • Alterations in cranial nerve function (V, VII, IX, X, XII) • Dry mouth • Oral lesions interfering with eating ability • Impaired tongue movement • Ill-fitting dentures or broken dentures

Biting/Chewing (Masticatory) Difficulty (NC-1.2)

Food/Nutrition-Related History	Reports or observations of: • Decreased estimated food intake • Alterations in estimated food intake from usual • Decreased estimated intake or avoidance of food difficult to form into a bolus, e.g., nuts, whole pieces of meat, poultry, fish, fruits, vegetables • Avoidance of foods of age-appropriate texture • Spitting food out or prolonged feeding time
Client History	• Conditions associated with a diagnosis or treatment, e.g., alcoholism; Alzheimer's; head, neck or pharyngeal cancer; cerebral palsy; cleft lip/palate; oral soft tissue infections (e.g., candidiasis, leukoplakia); lack of developmental readiness; oral manifestations of systemic disease (e.g., rheumatoid arthritis, lupus, Crohn's disease, penphigus vulgaris, HIV, diabetes) • Recent major oral surgery • Wired jaw • Chemotherapy with oral side effects • Radiation therapy to oral cavity

DIAGNOSIS

Updated: 2008 Edition

Breastfeeding Difficulty (NC-1.3)

Definition
Inability to sustain infant nutrition through breastfeeding.

Etiology (Cause/Contributing Risk Factors)
Factors gathered during the nutrition assessment process that contribute to the existence or the maintenance of pathophysiological, psychosocial, situational, developmental, cultural, and/or environmental problems:

Infant:
- Difficulty latching on, e.g., tight frenulum
- Poor sucking ability
- Oral pain
- Malnutrition/malabsorption
- Lethargy, sleepiness
- Irritability
- Swallowing difficulty
- Introduction of feeding via bottle or other route that may affect breastfeeding

Mother:
- Painful breasts, nipples
- Breast or nipple abnormality
- Mastitis
- Perception of or actual inadequate breastmilk* supply
- Lack of social or environmental support
- Cultural practices that affect the ability to breastfeed
- Introduction of feeding via bottle or other route that may affect breastfeeding

Signs/Symptoms (Defining Characteristics)
A typical cluster of subjective and objective signs and symptoms gathered during the nutrition assessment process that provide evidence that a problem exists; quantify the problem and describe its severity.

Nutrition Assessment Category	Potential Indicators of This Nutrition Diagnosis (one or more must be present)
Biochemical Data, Medical Tests and Procedures	• Laboratory evidence of dehydration (infant) • Fewer than reference standard, e.g., six wet diapers in 24 hours (infant)
Anthropometric Measurements	• Any weight loss or poor weight gain (infant)
Nutrition-Focused Physical Findings	• Frenulum abnormality (infant) • Vomiting or diarrhea (infant) • Hunger, lack of satiety after feeding (infant)

*If a synonym for the term "breastmilk" is helpful or needed, an approved alternate is "human milk."

238

Breastfeeding Difficulty (NC-1.3)

Food/Nutrition-Related History	Reports or observations of (infant): • Coughing • Crying, latching on and off, pounding on breasts • Decreased feeding frequency/duration, early cessation of feeding, and/or feeding resistance • Lethargy Reports or observations of (mother): • Small amount of breastmilk* when pumping • Lack of confidence in ability to breastfeed • Doesn't hear infant swallowing • Concerns regarding mother's choice to breastfeed/lack of support • Insufficient knowledge of breastfeeding or infant hunger/satiety signals • Lack of facilities or accommodations at place of employment or in community for breastfeeding • Feeding via bottle or other route
Client History	• Conditions associated with a diagnosis or treatment (infant), e.g., cleft lip/palate, thrush, premature birth, malabsorption, infection • Conditions associated with a diagnosis or treatment (mother), e.g., mastitis, candidiasis, engorgement, history of breast surgery

Updated: 2013 Edition

DIAGNOSIS

4th Edition

Altered Gastrointestinal (GI) Function (NC-1.4)

Definition
Changes in digestion, absorption, or elimination.

Etiology (Cause/Contributing Risk Factors)
Factors gathered during the nutrition assessment process that contribute to the existence or the maintenance of pathophysiological, psychosocial, situational, developmental, cultural, and/or environmental problems:

- Alteration in gastrointestinal tract structure and/or function
- Changes in the GI tract motility, e.g., gastroparesis
- Compromised exocrine function of related GI organs, e.g., pancreas, liver
- Decreased functional length of the GI tract, e.g., short-bowel syndrome

Signs/Symptoms (Defining Characteristics)
A typical cluster of subjective and objective signs and symptoms gathered during the nutrition assessment process that provide evidence that a problem exists; quantify the problem and describe its severity.

Nutrition Assessment Category	Potential Indicators of This Nutrition Diagnosis (one or more must be present)
Biochemical Data, Medical Tests and Procedures	• Abnormal digestive enzyme and fecal fat studies • Abnormal hydrogen breath test, d-xylose test, stool culture, and gastric emptying and/or small bowel transit time • Endoscopic or colonoscopic examination results, biopsy results • Abnormal anemia profile • Abnormal vitamin, mineral, fatty acid, trace element, and PTH results
Anthropometric Measurements	• Weight loss of ≥ 5% in one month, ≥ 10% in six months • Growth stunting or failure in children • Abnormal bone mineral density tests
Nutrition-Focused Physical Findings	• Abdominal distension • Increased (or sometimes decreased) bowel sounds • Wasting due to malnutrition in severe cases • Anorexia, nausea, vomiting, diarrhea, steatorrhea, constipation, abdominal pain, reflux, gas • Evidence of vitamin and/or mineral deficiency, e.g., glossitis, cheilosis, mouth lesions, skin rashes, hair loss

DIAGNOSIS

Altered Gastrointestinal (GI) Function (NC-1.4)

Food/Nutrition-Related History	Reports or observations of: • Avoidance or limitation of estimated total intake or intake of specific foods/food groups due to GI symptoms, e.g., bloating, cramping, pain, diarrhea, steatorrhea (greasy, floating, foul-smelling stools) especially following ingestion of food
Client History	• Conditions associated with a diagnosis or treatment, e.g., malabsorption, maldigestion, steatorrhea, obstruction, constipation, diverticulitis, Crohn's disease, inflammatory bowel disease, cystic fibrosis, celiac disease, cancers, irritable bowel syndrome, infection, dumping syndrome • Surgical procedures, e.g., esophagectomy, dilatation, fundoplication, gastrectomy, vagotomy, gastric bypass, bowel resections

Updated: 2011 Edition

DIAGNOSIS

Impaired Nutrient Utilization (NC-2.1)

Definition

Changes in ability to metabolize nutrients and bioactive substances.

Etiology (Cause/Contributing Risk Factors)

Factors gathered during the nutrition assessment process that contribute to the existence or the maintenance of pathophysiological, psychosocial, situational, developmental, cultural, and/or environmental problems:

- Compromised endocrine function of related GI organs, e.g., pancreas, liver, pituitary, parathyroid
- Metabolic disorders, including inborn errors of metabolism
- Medications that affect nutrient metabolism
- Alcohol or drug addiction

Signs/Symptoms (Defining Characteristics)

A typical cluster of subjective and objective signs and symptoms gathered during the nutrition assessment process that provide evidence that a problem exists; quantify the problem and describe its severity.

Nutrition Assessment Category	Potential Indicators of This Nutrition Diagnosis (one or more must be present)
Biochemical Data, Medical Tests and Procedures	• Abnormal tests for inborn errors of metabolism • Abnormal liver function tests • Abnormal anemia profile • Abnormal pituitary hormones (growth hormone [GH], adrenocorticotropic hormone [ACTH], luteinizing hormone [LH] and follicle-stimulating hormone [FSH]) • Vitamin and/or mineral deficiency • Hypoglycemia, hyperglycemia • Abnormal PTH
Anthropometric Measurements	• Weight loss of $\geq$ 5% in one month, $\geq$ 10% in six months • Growth stunting or failure in children • Abnormal bone mineral density tests
Nutrition-Focused Physical Findings	• Evidence of vitamin and/or mineral deficiency, e.g., glossitis, cheilosis, mouth lesions • Thin, wasted appearance
Food/Nutrition-Related History	Reports or observations of: • Avoidance or limitation of intake of specific foods/food groups due to physical symptoms • Alcohol or drug use

Impaired Nutrient Utilization (NC-2.1)

Client History	• Conditions associated with a diagnosis or treatment, e.g., cystic fibrosis, celiac disease, Crohn's disease, infection, radiation therapy, inborn errors of metabolism, endocrine disorders, pituitary disorders, renal failure, liver failure

Updated: 2013 Edition

DIAGNOSIS

Altered Nutrition-Related Laboratory Values (Specify) (NC-2.2)

Definition
Changes due to body composition, medications, body system changes or genetics, or changes in ability to eliminate byproducts of digestive and metabolic processes.

Etiology (Cause/Contributing Risk Factors)
Factors gathered during the nutrition assessment process that contribute to the existence or the maintenance of pathophysiological, psychosocial, situational, developmental, cultural, and/or environmental problems:

- Kidney, liver, cardiac, endocrine, neurologic, and/or pulmonary dysfunction
- Prematurity
- Other organ dysfunction that leads to biochemical changes

Signs/Symptoms (Defining Characteristics)
A typical cluster of subjective and objective signs and symptoms gathered during the nutrition assessment process that provide evidence that a problem exists; quantify the problem and describe its severity.

Nutrition Assessment Category	Potential Indicators of This Nutrition Diagnosis (one or more must be present)
Biochemical Data, Medical Tests and Procedures	• ↑ AST, ALT, T. bili, serum ammonia (liver disorders) • ↑ BUN, ↑ Cr, ↑ K, ↑ phosphorus, ↓ glomerular filtration rate (GFR) (kidney disorders) • Altered pO_2 and pCO_2 (pulmonary disorders) • ↑ Serum lipids • ↑ Plasma glucose and/or HgbA1c levels • Inadequate blood glucose control • ↑ Urine microalbumin • Other findings of acute or chronic disorders that are abnormal and of nutritional origin or consequence
Anthropometric Measurements	• Rapid weight changes • Other anthropometric measures that are altered
Nutrition-Focused Physical Findings	• Jaundice, edema, ascites, pruritis (liver disorders) • Edema, shortness of breath (cardiac disorders) • Blue nail beds, clubbing (pulmonary disorders) • Anorexia, nausea, vomiting

Arrows used with laboratory values: ↑ represents above reference standard and ↓ represents below reference standard

Altered Nutrition-Related Laboratory Values (Specify) (NC-2.2)

Food/Nutrition-Related History	Reports or observations of: • Estimated intake of foods high in or overall excess intake of protein, potassium, phosphorus, sodium, fluid • Estimated intake of micronutrients less than recommendations • Food- and nutrition-related knowledge deficit, e.g., lack of information, incorrect information, or noncompliance with modified diet
Client History	• Conditions associated with a diagnosis or treatment, e.g., renal or liver disease, alcoholism, cardiopulmonary disorders, diabetes

Updated: 2013 Edition

DIAGNOSIS

Food–Medication Interaction (Specify) (NC-2.3)

Definition
Undesirable/harmful interaction(s) between food and over-the-counter (OTC) medications, prescribed medications, herbals, botanicals, and/or dietary supplements that diminishes, enhances, or alters the effect of nutrients and/or medications.

Etiology (Cause/Contributing Risk Factors)
Factors gathered during the nutrition assessment process that contribute to the existence or the maintenance of pathophysiological, psychosocial, situational, developmental, cultural, and/or environmental problems:

- Combined ingestion or administration of medication and food that results in undesirable/harmful interaction

Signs/Symptoms (Defining Characteristics)
A typical cluster of subjective and objective signs and symptoms gathered during the nutrition assessment process that provide evidence that a problem exists; quantify the problem and describe its severity.

Nutrition Assessment Category	Potential Indicators of This Nutrition Diagnosis (one or more must be present)
Biochemical Data, Medical Tests and Procedures	• Alterations of biochemical tests based on medication affect and patient/client condition
Anthropometric Measurements	• Alterations of anthropometric measurements based on medication effect and patient/client conditions, e.g., weight gain and corticosteroids
Nutrition-Focused Physical Findings	• Changes in appetite or taste

DIAGNOSIS

Food–Medication Interaction (Specify) (NC-2.3)

Food/Nutrition-Related History	Reports or observations of:
	• Intake that is problematic or inconsistent with OTC, prescribed drugs, herbals, botanicals, or dietary supplements, such as:
	  ▪ fish oils and prolonged bleeding
	  ▪ coumadin and vitamin K-rich foods
	  ▪ high-fat diet while on cholesterol-lowering medications
	  ▪ iron supplements, constipation, and low-fiber diet
	• Intake that does not support replacement or mitigation of OTC, prescribed drugs, herbals, botanicals, and dietary supplements effects
	• Multiple drugs (OTC, prescribed drugs, herbals, botanicals, or dietary supplements) that are known to have food–medication interactions
	• Medications that require nutrient supplementation that can not be accomplished via food intake, e.g., isoniazid and vitamin B-6

Client History	

DIAGNOSIS

Predicted Food–Medication Interaction (Specify) (NC-2.4)

Definition

Potential undesirable/harmful interaction(s) between food and over-the-counter (OTC) medications, prescribed medications, herbals, botanicals, and/or dietary supplements that diminishes, enhances, or alters the effect of nutrients and/or medications.

> Note: Appropriate nutrition diagnosis when food–medication interaction is predicted, but has not yet occurred. This nutrition diagnosis is used when the practitioner wants to prevent a nutrient-medication interaction. Observed food–medication interactions should be documented using Food–Medication Interaction (NC-2.3.1).

Etiology (Cause/Contributing Risk Factors)

Factors gathered during the nutrition assessment process that contribute to the existence or the maintenance of pathophysiological, psychosocial, situational, developmental, cultural, and/or environmental problems:

- Combined ingestion or administration of medication and food that results in undesirable/harmful interaction

Signs/Symptoms (Defining Characteristics)

A typical cluster of subjective and objective signs and symptoms gathered during the nutrition assessment process that provide evidence that a problem exists; quantify the problem and describe its severity.

Nutrition Assessment Category	Potential Indicators of This Nutrition Diagnosis (one or more must be present)
Biochemical Data, Medical Tests and Procedures	
Anthropometric Measurements	
Nutrition-Focused Physical Findings	

Predicted Food–Medication Interaction (Specify) (NC-2.4)

Food/Nutrition-Related History	Reports or observations of:
	 • Intake that is expected to be problematic or inconsistent with OTC, prescribed drugs, herbals, botanicals, or dietary supplements, such as:
	     ▪ fish oils and prolonged bleeding
	     ▪ coumadin and vitamin K-rich foods
	     ▪ high-fat diet while on cholesterol-lowering medications
	     ▪ iron supplements, constipation, and low-fiber diet
	 • Intake that may not support replacement or mitigation of OTC, prescribed drugs, herbals, botanicals, and dietary supplements effects
	 • Multiple drugs (OTC, prescribed drugs, herbals, botanicals, or dietary supplements) that are known to have food–medication interactions
	 • Medications that require nutrient supplementation that can not be accomplished via food intake, e.g., isoniazid and vitamin B-6

Client History	

DIAGNOSIS

Created: 2011 Edition

Underweight (NC-3.1)

Definition
Low body weight compared to established reference standards or recommendations.

Etiology (Cause/Contributing Risk Factors)
Factors gathered during the nutrition assessment process that contribute to the existence or the maintenance of pathophysiological, psychosocial, situational, developmental, cultural, and/or environmental problems:

- Disordered eating pattern
- Excessive physical activity
- Unsupported beliefs/attitudes about food, nutrition, and nutrition-related topics
- Inadequate energy intake
- Increased energy needs
- Lack of or limited access to food
- Small for gestational age, intrauterine growth retardation/restriction and/or lack of progress/appropriate weight gain per day

Signs/Symptoms (Defining Characteristics)
A typical cluster of subjective and objective signs and symptoms gathered during the nutrition assessment process that provide evidence that a problem exists; quantify the problem and describe its severity.

Nutrition Assessment Category	Potential Indicators of This Nutrition Diagnosis (one or more must be present)
Biochemical Data, Medical Tests and Procedures	• ↑ Measured resting metabolic rate (RMR) higher than expected and/or estimated

Anthropometric Measurements	• Decreased skinfold thickness and mid-arm muscle circumference
	• BMI < 18.5 (adults)
	• BMI for older adults (older than 65 years) < 23
	• Birth to 2 years
	  ▪ Weight for age < 5th percentile
	  ▪ Weight for length < 5th percentile
	• Ages 2 to 20 years
	  ▪ Weight for stature < 5th percentile
	  ▪ BMI < 5th percentile (for children 2 to 20)
	  ▪ Weight for age < 5th percentile

Nutrition-Focused Physical Findings	• Decreased muscle mass, muscle wasting (gluteal and temporal) • Hunger

Arrows used with laboratory values: ↑ represents above reference standard and ↓ represents below reference standard

Underweight (NC-3.1)

Food/Nutrition-Related History	Reports or observations of: • Estimated intake of food less than estimated or measured needs • Limited supply of food in home • Dieting, food faddism • Refusal to eat • Physical activity more than recommended amount • Medications that affect appetite, e.g., stimulants for ADHD
Client History	• Malnutrition • Illness or physical disability • Mental illness, dementia, confusion • Athlete, dancer, gymnast • Vitamin/mineral deficiency

Updated: 2013 Edition

DIAGNOSIS

4th Edition

Unintended* Weight Loss (NC-3.2)

Definition
Decrease in body weight that is not planned or desired.

> *Note:May not be an appropriate nutrition diagnosis when changes in body weight are due to fluid.*

Etiology (Cause/Contributing Risk Factors)
Factors gathered during the nutrition assessment process that contribute to the existence or the maintenance of pathophysiological, psychosocial, situational, developmental, cultural, and/or environmental problems:

- Physiological causes increasing nutrient needs, e.g., due to prolonged catabolic illness, trauma, malabsorption
- Decreased ability to consume sufficient energy
- Lack of or limited access to food, e.g., economic constraints, restricting food given to elderly and/or children
- Cultural practices that affect ability to access food
- Prolonged hospitalization
- Psychological causes such as depression and disordered eating
- Lack of self-feeding ability

Signs/Symptoms (Defining Characteristics)
A typical cluster of subjective and objective signs and symptoms gathered during the nutrition assessment process that provide evidence that a problem exists; quantify the problem and describe its severity.

Nutrition Assessment Category	Potential Indicators of This Nutrition Diagnosis (one or more must be present)
Biochemical Data, Medical Tests and Procedures	
Anthropometric Measurements	• Weight loss of ≥ 5% within 30 days, ≥ 7.5% in 90 days, or ≥ 10% in 180 days (adults) • Not gaining weight as expected; 5% weight loss in 6 months and/or a shift downward in growth percentiles, crossing two or more percentile channels on reference growth standard charts (pediatrics)

*If a synonym, or alternate word with the same meaning, for the term "unintended" is helpful or needed, an approved alternate is the word "involuntary."

Unintended* Weight Loss (NC-3.2)

Nutrition-Focused Physical Findings	• Fever • Decreased senses, i.e., smell, taste, vision • Increased heart rate • Increased respiratory rate • Loss of subcutaneous fat and muscle stores • Change in way clothes fit • Changes in mental status or function (e.g., depression)
Food/Nutrition-Related History	Reports or observations of: • Normal or usual estimated intake in face of illness • Poor intake, change in eating habits, early satiety, skipped meals • Medications associated with weight loss, such as certain antidepressants
Client History	• Conditions associated with a diagnosis or treatment, e.g., AIDS/HIV, burns, chronic obstructive pulmonary disease, dysphagia, hip/long bone fracture, infection, surgery, trauma, hyperthyroidism (pre- or untreated), some types of cancer or metastatic disease (specify), substance abuse • Cancer chemotherapy

DIAGNOSIS

Updated: 2013 Edition

*If a synonym, or alternate word with the same meaning, for the term "unintended" is helpful or needed, an approved alternate is the word "involuntary."

4th Edition

Overweight/Obesity (NC-3.3)

Definition
Increased adiposity compared to established reference standards or recommendations, ranging from overweight to morbid obesity.

Etiology (Cause/Contributing Risk Factors)
Factors gathered during the nutrition assessment process that contribute to the existence or the maintenance of pathophysiological, psychosocial, situational, developmental, cultural, and/or environmental problems:

- Decreased energy needs
- Disordered eating pattern
- Excessive energy intake
- Food- and nutrition-related knowledge deficit
- Not ready for diet/lifestyle change
- Physical inactivity
- Increased psychological/life stress

Signs/Symptoms (Defining Characteristics)
A typical cluster of subjective and objective signs and symptoms gathered during the nutrition assessment process that provide evidence that a problem exists; quantify the problem and describe its severity.

Nutrition Assessment Category	Potential Indicators of This Nutrition Diagnosis (one or more must be present)
Biochemical Data, Medical Tests and Procedures	• ↓ Measured resting metabolic rate (RMR) less than expected and/or estimated

Anthropometric Measurements	• BMI more than normative standard for age and sex:
	  ▪ Overweight: 25 to 29.9 (adults), 85th to 94th percentiles (pediatrics)
	  ▪ Obese Class I: 30 to 34.9 (adults)
	  ▪ Obese Class II: 35 to 39.9 (adults)
	  ▪ Obese Class III: 40+* (adults)
	  ▪ Obese > 95th percentile (pediatrics)
	• Waist circumference more than normative standard for age and sex
	• Increased skinfold thickness
	• Body fat percentage >25% for men and >32% for women
	• Weight for height more than normative standard for age and sex

Arrows used with laboratory values: ↑ represents above reference standard and ↓ represents below reference standard.

*If a synonym for the term "Obese Class III" is helpful or needed, an approved alternate is "morbid obesity."

Overweight/Obesity (NC-3.3)

Nutrition-Focused Physical Findings	• Increased body adiposity
Food/Nutrition-Related History	Reports or observations of: • Overconsumption of high-fat and/or energy-dense food or beverage • Large portions of food (portion size more than twice than recommended) • Estimated excessive energy intake • Infrequent, low-duration and/or low-intensity physical activity, factors affecting physical activity access • Large amounts of sedentary activities, e.g., TV watching, reading, computer use in both leisure and work/school • Uncertainty regarding nutrition-related recommendations • Inability to apply nutrition-related recommendations • Unwillingness or disinterest in applying nutrition-related recommendations • Inability to lose a significant amount of excess weight through conventional weight loss intervention • Medications that impact RMR, e.g., midazolam, propranolol, glipizide
Client History	• Conditions associated with a diagnosis or treatment, e.g., hypothyroidism, metabolic syndrome, eating disorder not otherwise specified, depression • Physical disability or limitation • History of familial obesity • History of childhood obesity • History of physical, sexual, or emotional abuse

DIAGNOSIS

Updated: 2013 Edition

Unintended* Weight Gain (NC-3.4)

Definition
Weight gain more than that which is desired or planned.

Etiology (Cause/Contributing Risk Factors)
Factors gathered during the nutrition assessment process that contribute to the existence or the maintenance of pathophysiological, psychosocial, situational, developmental, cultural, and/or environmental problems:
- Illness causing unexpected weight gain because of head trauma, immobility, paralysis or related condition
- Chronic use of medications known to cause weight gain, such as use of certain antidepressants, antipsycho-tics, corticosteroids, certain HIV medications
- Condition leading to excessive fluid weight gains

Signs/Symptoms (Defining Characteristics)
A typical cluster of subjective and objective signs and symptoms gathered during the nutrition assessment process that provide evidence that a problem exists; quantify the problem and describe its severity.

Nutrition Assessment Category	Potential Indicators of This Nutrition Diagnosis (one or more must be present)
Biochemical Data, Medical Tests and Procedures	• ↓ Serum albumin, hyponatremia, ↑ fasting serum lipid levels, ↑ fasting glucose levels, fluctuating hormone levels
Anthropometric Measurements	• Increased weight, any increase in weight more than planned or desired (pediatrics and adults) • Grams/day > than planned or desired (pediatrics) • Weight gain of > 5% within 30 days, > 7.5% in 90 days, or > 10% in 180 days (adults)
Nutrition-Focused Physical Findings	• Fat accumulation, excessive subcutaneous fat stores, noticeable change in body fat distribution • Extreme hunger with or without palpitations, tremor, and sweating • Edema • Shortness of breath • Muscle weakness • Fatigue

Arrows used with laboratory values: ↑ represents above reference standard and ↓ represents below reference standard.

If a synonym, or alternate word with the same meaning, for the term "unintended" is helpful or needed, an approved alternate is the word "involuntary."

Unintended* Weight Gain (NC-3.4)

Food/Nutrition-Related History	Reports or observations of: • Estimated intake inconsistent with estimated or measured energy needs • Changes in recent estimated food intake level • Fluid administration more than requirements • Use of alcohol, narcotics • Medications associated with increased appetite • Physical inactivity or change in physical activity level
Client History	• Conditions associated with a diagnosis or treatment of asthma, psychiatric illnesses, rheumatic conditions, Cushing's syndrome, obesity, Prader-Willi syndrome, hypothyroidism

pdated: 2013 Edition

DIAGNOSIS

f a synonym, or alternate word with the same meaning, for the term "unintended" is helpful or eeded, an approved alternate is the word "involuntary."

4th Edition

Suboptimal Growth Rate (NC-3.5)

Definition
Rate of growth or growth velocity slower than expected, or weight gain that is suboptimal in comparison with goal or reference standard.

Etiology (Cause/Contributing Risk Factors)
Factors gathered during the nutrition assessment process that contribute to the existence of or the maintenance of pathophysiological, psychosocial, situational, developmental, cultural, and/or environmental problems.

- Physiological impetus for increased nutrient needs (e.g., critical illness or trauma; pregnancy; metabolic illness, e.g., type 1 diabetes; malabsorption)
- Decreased ability to consume sufficient energy
- Lack of or limited access to food
- Psychological causes, such as depression or disordered eating pattern
- Limited food acceptance
- Food and nutrition-related knowledge deficit
- Unsupported beliefs/attitudes about food, nutrition, and nutrition-related topics
- Small for gestational age, intrauterine growth restriction/retardation, lack of appropriate weight gain, hyperemesis gravidarum

Signs/Symptoms (Defining Characteristics)
A typical cluster of subjective and objective signs and symptoms gathered during the nutrition assessment process that provide evidence that a problem exists; quantify the problem and describe its severity.

Nutrition Assessment Category	Potential Indicators of This Nutrition Diagnosis (one or more must be present)
Biochemical Data, Medical Tests and Procedures	• Positive urine ketones, ↑ fasting (or postprandial) glucose level • Fluctuating hormone levels during pregnancy • Zinc deficiency • Iron deficiency
Anthropometric Measurements	• Weight-for-age decrease in 2 or more percentile channels • Weight-gain velocity less than expected, based on established reference standard and/or guideline • Length- or height-for-age decrease in 2 or more percentile channels • Length- or height-gain velocity less than expected, based on established reference standard and/or guideline

Arrows used with laboratory values: ↑ represents above reference standard and ↓ represents below reference standard.

Suboptimal Growth Rate (NC-3.5)

Nutrition-Focused Physical Findings	• Decreased muscle mass, muscle wasting (gluteal and temporal) • Hunger • Decreased fat mass
Food/Nutrition-Related History	Reports or observations of: • Estimated energy intake inconsistent with estimated or measured needs. • Restricted fluids decreasing ability to meet nutritional needs • Difficulty breastfeeding, e.g., poor latch • Limited food acceptance, e.g., not progressing to foods as expected or recommended • Medications associated with decreased appetite or weight loss • Use of alcohol or narcotics during pregnancy • Increase in physical activity levels • Normal or usual intake in presence of illness • Poor intake, change in eating habits, early satiety, or skipped meals
Client History	• Conditions associated with a diagnosis or treatment impacting growth, including AIDS/HIV, burns, pulmonary disease, dysphagia, long bone fracture, infection, surgery, trauma, hyperthyroid, hypothyroid, substance abuse, some types of cancer or metastatic disease. • Food insecurity

DIAGNOSIS

Created: 2013 Edition

Excessive Growth Rate (NC-3.6)

Definition
Rate of growth or growth velocity greater than expected, or weight gain that is higher in comparison with goal or reference standard.

Etiology (Cause/Contributing Risk Factors)
Factors gathered during the nutrition assessment process that contribute to the existence of or the maintenance of pathophysiological, psychosocial, situational, developmental, cultural, and/or environmental problems.

- Physiological change resulting in decreased energy needs
- Excessive energy intake
- Frequent intake of energy-dense foods
- Food and nutrition-related knowledge deficit
- Physical inactivity

Signs/Symptoms (Defining Characteristics)
A typical cluster of subjective and objective signs and symptoms gathered during the nutrition assessment process that provide evidence that a problem exists; quantify the problem and describe its severity.

Nutrition Assessment Category	Potential Indicators of This Nutrition Diagnosis (one or more must be present)
Biochemical Data, Medical Tests and Procedures	
Anthropometric Measurements	• Weight gain greater than reference standard • Weight gain velocity greater than expected, based on reference standard and/or guidelines • Weight-for-length or BMI-for-age increase greater than expected
Nutrition-Focused Physical Findings	
Food/Nutrition-Related History	Reports or observations of: • Estimated energy intake inconsistent with estimated or measured needs • Medications associated with increased appetite or weight gain • Decrease in physical activity
Client History	• Conditions associated with a diagnosis or treatment impacting growth, e.g., Prader-Willi syndrome, Down syndrome, spina bifida, and neurological conditions that impact satiety

Created: 2013 Edition

Food- and Nutrition-Related Knowledge Deficit (NB-1.1)

Definition
Incomplete or inaccurate knowledge about food, nutrition, or nutrition-related information and guidelines.

Etiology (Cause/Contributing Risk Factors)
Factors gathered during the nutrition assessment process that contribute to the existence or the maintenance of pathophysiological, psychosocial, situational, developmental, cultural, and/or environmental problems:

- Unsupported beliefs/attitudes about food, nutrition, and nutrition-related topics
- Lack of prior nutrition-related education
- Lack of understanding of infant/child cues to indicate hunger
- Cultural beliefs that affect ability to learn/apply information
- Impaired cognitive ability, including learning disabilities, neurological or sensory impairment, and/or dementia
- Prior exposure to incorrect information
- Unwilling or disinterested in learning/applying information
- Uncertainty how to apply nutrition information

Signs/Symptoms (Defining Characteristics)
A typical cluster of subjective and objective signs and symptoms gathered during the nutrition assessment process that provide evidence that a problem exists; quantify the problem and describe its severity.

Nutrition Assessment Category	Potential Indicators of This Nutrition Diagnosis (one or more must be present)
Biochemical Data, Medical Tests and Procedures	
Anthropometric Measurements	
Nutrition-Focused Physical Findings	

4th Edition

Food- and Nutrition-Related Knowledge Deficit (NB-1.1)

Food/Nutrition-Related History	Reports or observations of: • Verbalizes inaccurate or incomplete information • Provides inaccurate or incomplete written response to questionnaire/written tool or is unable to read written tool • No prior knowledge of need for food- and nutrition-related recommendations • No prior education provided on how to apply food and nutrition related information • Demonstrates inability to apply food- and nutrition-related information, e.g., select food based on nutrition therapy or prepare infant feeding as instructed • Relates concerns about previous attempts to learn information • Verbalizes unwillingness or disinterest in learning information
Client History	• Conditions associated with a diagnosis or treatment • New medical diagnosis or change in existing diagnosis or condition • Ethnic or cultural related issues impacting application of information

Updated: 2013 Edition

Unsupported Beliefs/Attitudes About Food or Nutrition-Related Topics (NB-1.2)

Use with caution: Be sensitive to patient/client concerns.

Definition

Beliefs/attitudes or practices about food, nutrition, and nutrition-related topics that are incompatible with sound nutrition principles, nutrition care, or disease/condition (excluding disordered eating patterns and eating disorders).

Etiology (Cause/Contributing Risk Factors)

Factors gathered during the nutrition assessment process that contribute to the existence or the maintenance of pathophysiological, psychosocial, situational, developmental, cultural, and/or environmental problems:

- Disbelief in science-based food and nutrition information
- Lack of prior exposure to accurate nutrition-related information
- Eating behavior serves a purpose other than nourishment (e.g., pica)
- Desire for a cure for a chronic disease through the use of alternative therapy

Signs/Symptoms (Defining Characteristics)

A typical cluster of subjective and objective signs and symptoms gathered during the nutrition assessment process that provide evidence that a problem exists; quantify the problem and describe its severity.

Nutrition Assessment Category	Potential Indicators of This Nutrition Diagnosis (one or more must be present)
Biochemical Data, Medical Tests and Procedures	
Anthropometric Measurements	
Nutrition-Focused Physical Findings	
Food/Nutrition-Related History	Reports or observations of: • Food faddism • Estimated intake that reflects an imbalance of nutrients/food groups • Avoidance of foods/food groups (e.g., sugar, wheat, cooked foods) • Intake of nonfood items • Intake of complementary and alternative medicine products and dietary supplements that may be unsupported for health

Unsupported Beliefs/Attitudes About Food or Nutrition-Related Topics (NB-1.2)

Use with caution: Be sensitive to patient/client concerns.

Client History	• Conditions associated with a diagnosis or treatment, e.g., obesity, diabetes, cancer, cardiovascular disease, mental illness • Pica • Food fetish

Updated: 2013 Edition

Not Ready for Diet/Lifestyle Change (NB-1.3)

Definition

Lack of perceived value of nutrition-related behavior change compared to costs (consequences or effort required to make changes); conflict with personal value system; preceding event, condition or cause to behavior change.

Etiology (Cause/Contributing Risk Factors)

Factors gathered during the nutrition assessment process that contribute to the existence or the maintenance of pathophysiological, psychosocial, situational, developmental, cultural, and/or environmental problems:

- Unsupported beliefs/attitudes about food, nutrition, and nutrition-related topics
- Impaired cognitive ability, including learning disabilities, neurological or sensory impairment, and/or dementia
- Lack of social support for implementing changes
- Denial of need to change
- Perception that time, interpersonal, or financial constraints prevent changes
- Unwilling or disinterested in learning/applying information
- Lack of self-efficacy for making change or demoralization from previous failures at change

Signs/Symptoms (Defining Characteristics)

A typical cluster of subjective and objective signs and symptoms gathered during the nutrition assessment process that provide evidence that a problem exists; quantify the problem and describe its severity.

Nutrition Assessment Category	Potential Indicators of This Nutrition Diagnosis (one or more must be present)
Biochemical Data, Medical Tests and Procedures	
Anthropometric Measurements	
Nutrition-Focused Physical Findings	• Negative body language, e.g., frowning, lack of eye contact, defensive posture, lack of focus, fidgeting (Note: body language varies by culture.)

DIAGNOSIS

Not Ready for Diet/Lifestyle Change (NB-1.3)

Food/Nutrition-Related History	Reports or observations of: • Denial of need for food- and nutrition-related changes • Inability to understand required changes • Failure to keep appointments/schedule follow-up appointments or engage in counseling • Previous failures to effectively change target behavior • Defensiveness, hostility, or resistance to change • Lack of efficacy to make change or to overcome barriers to change • Factors affecting physical activity access
Client History	

Updated: 2008 Edition

Self-Monitoring Deficit (NB-1.4)

Definition
Lack of data recording to track personal progress.

Etiology (Cause/Contributing Risk Factors)
Factors gathered during the nutrition assessment process that contribute to the existence or the maintenance of pathophysiological, psychosocial, situational, developmental, cultural, and/or environmental problems:

- Food- and nutrition-related knowledge deficit concerning self-monitoring
- Lack of social support for implementing changes
- Lack of value for behavior change or competing values
- Perception that lack of resources (e.g., time, financial, or interpersonal) prevent self-monitoring
- Cultural practices that affect the ability to track personal progress
- Impaired cognitive ability, including learning disabilities, neurological or sensory impairment, and/or dementia
- Prior exposure to incompatible information
- Not ready for diet/lifestyle change
- Unwilling or disinterested in tracking progress
- Lack of focus and attention to detail, difficulty with time management and/or organization

Signs/Symptoms (Defining Characteristics)
A typical cluster of subjective and objective signs and symptoms gathered during the nutrition assessment process that provide evidence that a problem exists; quantify the problem and describe its severity.

Nutrition Assessment Category	Potential Indicators of This Nutrition Diagnosis (one or more must be present)
Biochemical Data, Medical Tests and Procedures	• Recorded data inconsistent with biochemical data, e.g., estimated dietary intake is not consistent with biochemical data
Anthropometric Measurements	
Nutrition-Focused Physical Findings	

Self-Monitoring Deficit (NB-1.4)

Food/Nutrition-Related History	Reports or observations of: • Incomplete self-monitoring records, e.g., glucose, food, fluid intake, weight, physical activity, ostomy output records • Estimated food intake data inconsistent with weight status or growth pattern data • Embarrassment or anger regarding need for self-monitoring • Uncertainty of how to complete monitoring records • Uncertainty regarding changes that could/should be made in response to data in self-monitoring records • No self-management equipment, e.g., no blood glucose monitor, pedometer • Verbalizes inaccurate or incomplete knowledge • Cultural or religious practices that affect intake
Client History	• Diagnoses associated with self-monitoring, e.g., diabetes mellitus, obesity, new ostomy • New medical diagnosis or change in existing diagnosis or condition • Lack of social and/or familial support

Disordered Eating Pattern (NB-1.5)

Definition

Beliefs, attitudes, thoughts, and behaviors related to food, eating, and weight management, including classic eating disorders as well as less severe, similar conditions that negatively impact health.

> *Note: May not be an appropriate nutrition diagnosis for individuals with Limited food acceptance NI-2.9.*

Etiology (Cause/Contributing Risk Factors)

Factors gathered during the nutrition assessment process that contribute to the existence or the maintenance of pathophysiological, psychosocial, situational, developmental, cultural, and/or environmental problems:

- Familial, societal, biological/genetic, and/or environmental-related obsessive desire to be thin
- Weight regulation/preoccupation significantly influences self-esteem

Signs/Symptoms (Defining Characteristics)

A typical cluster of subjective and objective signs and symptoms gathered during the nutrition assessment process that provide evidence that a problem exists; quantify the problem and describe its severity.

Nutrition Assessment Category	Potential Indicators of This Nutrition Diagnosis (one or more must be present)
Biochemical Data, Medical Tests and Procedures	• ↓ Cholesterol, abnormal lipid profiles, hypoglycemia, hypokalemia (anorexia nervosa [AN]) • Hypokalemia and hypochloremic alkalosis (bulimia nervosa [BN]) • Hyponatremia, hypothyroid, elevated BUN (AN) • Urine positive for ketones (AN)
Anthropometric Measurements	• BMI < 17.5, arrested growth and development, failure to gain weight during period of expected growth, weight less than 85% of expected (AN) • BMI > 29 (eating disorder not otherwise specified [EDNOS]) • Significant weight fluctuation (BN)
Nutrition-Focused Physical Findings	• Severely depleted adipose and somatic protein stores (AN) • Lanugo hair formation on face and trunk, brittle listless hair, cyanosis of hands and feet, and dry skin (AN) • Normal or excess adipose and normal somatic protein stores (BN, EDNOS) • Damaged tooth enamel (BN)

Arrows used with laboratory values: ↑ represents above reference standard and ↓ represents below reference standard.

Disordered Eating Pattern (NB-1.5)

Nutrition-Focused Physical Findings, cont'd	• Enlarged parotid glands (BN) • Peripheral edema (BN) • Skeletal muscle loss (AN) • Low body temperature • Inability to concentrate (AN) • Positive Russell's Sign (BN) callous on back of hand from self-induced vomiting • Bradycardia (heart rate < 60 beats/min), hypotension (systolic < 90 mm HG), and orthostatic hypotension (AN) • Self-induced vomiting, diarrhea, bloating, constipation, and flatulence (BN); always cold (AN) • Muscle weakness, fatigue, dehydration (AN, BN) • Denial of hunger (AN)
Food/Nutrition-Related History	Reports or observations of: • Avoidance of food or energy-containing beverages (AN, BN) • Avoidance of social events at which food is served • Fear of foods or dysfunctional thoughts regarding food or food experiences (AN, BN) • Food and weight preoccupation (AN, BN) • Knowledgeable about current diet fad (AN, BN, EDNOS) • Fasting (AN, BN) • Estimated intake of larger quantity of food in a defined time period, a sense of lack of control over eating (BN, EDNOS) • Excessive physical activity (AN, BN, EDNOS) • Eating much more rapidly than normal, until feeling uncomfortably full, consuming large amounts of food when not feeling physically hungry; eating alone because of embarrassment, feeling very guilty after overeating (EDNOS) • Eats in private (AN, BN) • Irrational thoughts about food's affect on the body (AN, BN, EDNOS) • Pattern of chronic dieting • Excessive reliance on nutrition terming and preoccupation with nutrient content of foods

Disordered Eating Pattern (NB-1.5)

Food/Nutrition-Related History, cont'd	Reports or observations of: • Inflexibility with food selection • Misuse of laxatives, enemas, diuretics, stimulants, and/or metabolic enhancers (AN, BN) • Excessive use of condiments and food mixing
Client History	• Diagnosis, e.g., anorexia nervosa, bulimia nervosa, binge eating, eating disorder not otherwise specified, amenorrhea • History of mood and anxiety disorders (e.g., depression, obsessive/compulsive disorder [OCD]), personality disorders, substance abuse disorders • Family history of eating disorder, depression, OCD, anxiety disorders (AN, BN) • Irritability, depression (AN, BN) • Anemia • Leukopenia • Cardiac arrhythmias, bradycardia (AN, BN)

DIAGNOSIS

Updated: 2011 Edition

Limited Adherence to Nutrition-Related Recommendations (NB-1.6)

Definition
Lack of nutrition-related changes as per intervention agreed on by client or population.

Etiology (Cause/Contributing Risk Factors)
Factors gathered during the nutrition assessment process that contribute to the existence or the maintenance of pathophysiological, psychosocial, situational, developmental, cultural, and/or environmental problems:

- Lack of social support for implementing changes
- Lack of value for behavior change or competing values
- Lack of confidence in ability to change
- Perception that lack of resources (e.g., time, financial, or interpersonal) prevent changes
- Previous lack of success in making health-related changes
- Food and nutrition-related knowledge deficit concerning how to make nutrition-related changes
- Unwilling or disinterested in applying/learning information
- Unsupported beliefs or attitudes about food or nutrition-related topics

Signs/Symptoms (Defining Characteristics)
A typical cluster of subjective and objective signs and symptoms gathered during the nutrition assessment process that provide evidence that a problem exists; quantify the problem and describe its severity.

Nutrition Assessment Category	Potential Indicators of This Nutrition Diagnosis (one or more must be present)
Biochemical Data, Medical Tests and Procedures	• Expected laboratory outcomes are not achieved
Anthropometric Measurements	• Expected anthropometric outcomes are not achieved
Nutrition-Focused Physical Findings	• Negative body language, e.g., frowning, lack of eye contact, fidgeting, defensive posture, crying (Note: body language varies by culture)

Limited Adherence to Nutrition-Related Recommendations (NB-1.6)

Food/Nutrition-Related History	Reports or observations of: • Expected food/nutrition-related outcomes are not achieved • Inability to recall changes agreed upon • Failure to complete any agreed upon homework • Lack of compliance or inconsistent compliance with plan • Failure to keep appointments or schedule follow-up appointments • Lack of appreciation of the importance of making recommended nutrition-related changes • Uncertainty as to how to consistently apply food/nutrition information • Verbalizes frustration with attempts to apply food/nutrition information • Verbalizes previous failures to effectively change target behavior • Presence of a lack of self-efficacy or confidence to make changes • Notes internal and/or external barriers to change
Client History	• Lack of social and/or familial support

Updated: 2013 Edition

DIAGNOSIS

Undesirable Food Choices (NB-1.7)

Definition

Food and/or beverage choices that are inconsistent with dietary reference intake standards (e.g., Dietary Reference Intakes), national food guidelines (e.g., US Dietary Guidelines, MyPlate), diet quality index standards (e.g., Healthy Eating Index) or as defined in the nutrition prescription.

Etiology (Cause/Contributing Risk Factors)

Factors gathered during the nutrition assessment process that contribute to the existence or the maintenance of pathophysiological, psychosocial, situational, developmental, cultural, and/or environmental problems:

- Lack of prior exposure to accurate nutrition-related information
- Cultural practices that affect the ability to learn/apply information
- Impaired cognitive ability, including learning disabilities, neurological or sensory impairment, and/or dementia
- High level of fatigue or other side effect of medical, surgical, or radiological therapy
- Lack of or limited access to recommended foods
- Perception that lack of resources (e.g., time, financial, or interpersonal) prevent selection of food choices consistent with recommendations
- Food allergies and aversions impeding food choices consistent with guidelines
- Lacks motivation and/or readiness to apply or support systems change
- Unwilling or disinterested in learning/applying information
- Psychological causes such as depression and disordered eating

Signs/Symptoms (Defining Characteristics)

A typical cluster of subjective and objective signs and symptoms gathered during the nutrition assessment process that provide evidence that a problem exists; quantify the problem and describe its severity.

Nutrition Assessment Category	Potential Indicators of This Nutrition Diagnosis (one or more must be present)
Biochemical Data, Medical Tests and Procedures	• ↑ lipid panel
Anthropometric Measurements	
Nutrition-Focused Physical Findings	• Findings consistent with vitamin/mineral deficiency or excess

Arrows used with laboratory values: ↑ represents above reference standard and ↓ represents below reference standard.

Undesirable Food Choices (NB-1.7)

Food/Nutrition-Related History	Reports or observations of: • Estimated intake inconsistent with dietary reference intake standards (e.g., DRIs), national food guidelines (e.g., US Dietary Guidelines, MyPlate), diet quality index standards (e.g., Healthy Eating Index), or nutrition prescription • Inaccurate or incomplete understanding of the guidelines • Inability to apply guideline information • Inability to select (e.g., access), or unwillingness or disinterest in selecting, food consistent with the guidelines
Client History	• Conditions associated with a diagnosis or treatment, e.g., mental illness

Updated: 2013 Edition

DIAGNOSIS

Physical Inactivity (NB-2.1)

Definition
Low level of activity or sedentary behavior to the extent that it reduces energy expenditure and impacts health.

Etiology (Cause/Contributing Risk Factors)
Factors gathered during the nutrition assessment process that contribute to the existence or the maintenance of pathophysiological, psychosocial, situational, developmental, cultural, and/or environmental problems:

- Unsupported beliefs/attitudes about physical activity
- Injury, lifestyle change, condition (e.g., advanced stages of cardiovascular disease, obesity, kidney disease), physical disability or limitation that reduces physical activity or activities of daily living
- Food and nutrition-related knowledge deficit concerning health benefits of physical activity
- Lack of prior exposure to accurate nutrition-related information
- Lack of role models, e.g., for children
- Lack of social support for implementing changes
- Lack of or limited access to safe exercise environment and/or equipment
- Lack of value for behavior change or competing values
- Time constraints
- Financial constraints that may prevent sufficient level of activity (e.g., cost of equipment or shoes or club membership to gain access)

Signs/Symptoms (Defining Characteristics)
A typical cluster of subjective and objective signs and symptoms gathered during the nutrition assessment process that provide evidence that a problem exists; quantify the problem and describe its severity.

Nutrition Assessment Category	Potential Indicators of This Nutrition Diagnosis (one or more must be present)
Biochemical Data, Medical Tests and Procedures	
Anthropometric Measurements	• Obesity: BMI > 30 (adults), BMI > 95th percentile (pediatrics > 3 years)
Nutrition-Focused Physical Findings	• Excessive subcutaneous fat and low muscle mass

Physical Inactivity (NB-2.1)

Food/Nutrition-Related History	Reports or observations of: • Infrequent, low-duration and/or low-intensity physical activity • Large amounts of sedentary activities, e.g., TV watching, reading, computer use in both leisure and work/school • Low level of NEAT (non-exercise activity thermogenesis) expended by physical activities other than planned exercise, e.g., sitting, standing, walking, fidgeting • Low cardiorespiratory fitness and/or low muscle strength • Medications that cause somnolence and decreased cognition • Factors affecting physical activity access
Client History	• Medical diagnoses that may be associated with or result in decreased activity, e.g., arthritis, chronic fatigue syndrome, morbid obesity, knee surgery • Psychological diagnosis, e.g., depression, anxiety disorders

DIAGNOSIS

Updated: 2008 Edition

Excessive Physical Activity (NB-2.2)

Definition
Involuntary or voluntary physical activity or movement that interferes with energy needs, growth, or exceeds that which is necessary to achieve optimal health.

Etiology (Cause/Contributing Risk Factors)
Factors gathered during the nutrition assessment process that contribute to the existence or the maintenance of pathophysiological, psychosocial, situational, developmental, cultural, and/or environmental problems:

- Disordered eating
- Irrational beliefs/attitudes about food, nutrition, and fitness
- "Addictive" behaviors/personality

Signs/Symptoms (Defining Characteristics)
A typical cluster of subjective and objective signs and symptoms gathered during the nutrition assessment process that provide evidence that a problem exists; quantify the problem and describe its severity.

Nutrition Assessment Category	Potential Indicators of This Nutrition Diagnosis (one or more must be present)
Biochemical Data, Medical Tests and Procedures	• ↑ Liver enzymes, e.g., LDH, AST • Altered micronutrient status, e.g., ↓ serum ferritin, zinc, and insulin-like growth factor-binding protein • ↑ Hematocrit • Possibly ↑ cortisol levels
Anthropometric Measurements	• Weight loss, arrested growth and development, failure to gain weight during period of expected growth (related usually to disordered eating)
Nutrition-Focused Physical Findings	• Depleted adipose and somatic protein stores (related usually to disordered eating) • Chronic muscle soreness
Food/Nutrition-Related History	Reports or observations of: • Continued/repeated high levels of exercise exceeding levels necessary to improve health and/or athletic performance • Exercise daily without rest/rehabilitation days • Exercise while injured/sick • Forsaking family, job, social responsibilities to exercise • Overtraining

Arrows used with laboratory values: ↑ represents above reference standard and ↓ represents below reference standard.

DIAGNOSIS

Excessive Physical Activity (NB-2.2)

Client History	• Conditions associated with a diagnosis or treatment, e.g., anorexia nervosa, bulimia nervosa, binge eating, eating disorder not otherwise specified, amenorrhea, stress fractures
	• Chronic fatigue
	• Evidence of addictive, obsessive, or compulsive tendencies
	• Suppressed immune function
	• Frequent and/or prolonged injuries and/or illnesses

Updated: 2009 Edition

DIAGNOSIS

Inability to Manage Self-Care (NB-2.3)

Definition
Lack of capacity or unwillingness to implement methods to support healthful food- and nutrition-related behavior.

Etiology (Cause/Contributing Risk Factors)
Factors gathered during the nutrition assessment process that contribute to the existence or the maintenance of pathophysiological, psychosocial, situational, developmental, cultural, and/or environmental problems:

- Food- and nutrition-related knowledge deficit concerning self-care
- Lack of social support for implementing changes
- Lack of developmental readiness to perform self-management tasks, e.g., pediatrics
- Lack of value for behavior change or competing values
- Perception that lack of resources (e.g., time, financial, or interpersonal) prevent self-care
- Cultural practices that affect ability to manage self-care
- Impaired cognitive ability, including learning disabilities, neurological or sensory impairment, and/or dementia
- Prior exposure to incompatible information
- Not ready for diet/lifestyle change
- Unwilling or disinterested in learning/applying information
- Lack of or limited access to self-management tools or decision guides

Signs/Symptoms (Defining Characteristics)
A typical cluster of subjective and objective signs and symptoms gathered during the nutrition assessment process that provide evidence that a problem exists; quantify the problem and describe its severity.

Nutrition Assessment Category	Potential Indicators of This Nutrition Diagnosis (one or more must be present)
Biochemical Data, Medical Tests and Procedures	
Anthropometric Measurements	
Nutrition-Focused Physical Findings	

Inability to Manage Self-Care (NB-2.3)

Food/Nutrition-Related History	Reports or observations of: • Inability to interpret data or self-management tools • Embarrassment or anger regarding need for self-monitoring • Uncertainty regarding changes could/should be made in response to data in self-monitoring records
Client History	• Diagnoses that are associated with self-management, e.g., diabetes mellitus, obesity, cardiovascular disease, renal or liver disease • Conditions associated with a diagnosis or treatment, e.g., cognitive or emotional impairment • New medical diagnosis or change in existing diagnosis or condition

Updated: 2013 Edition

DIAGNOSIS

Impaired Ability to Prepare Foods/ Meals (NB-2.4)

Definition
Cognitive or physical impairment that prevents preparation of foods/fluids.

Etiology (Cause/Contributing Risk Factors)
Factors gathered during the nutrition assessment process that contribute to the existence or the maintenance of pathophysiological, psychosocial, situational, developmental, cultural, and/or environmental problems:

- Impaired cognitive ability, including learning disabilities, neurological or sensory impairment, and/or dementia
- Loss of mental or cognitive ability, e.g., dementia
- Physical disability
- High level of fatigue or other side effect of therapy

Signs/Symptoms (Defining Characteristics)
A typical cluster of subjective and objective signs and symptoms gathered during the nutrition assessment process that provide evidence that a problem exists; quantify the problem and describe its severity.

Nutrition Assessment Category	Potential Indicators of This Nutrition Diagnosis (one or more must be present)
Biochemical Data, Medical Tests and Procedures	
Anthropometric Measurements	
Nutrition-Focused Physical Findings	
Food/Nutrition-Related History	Reports or observations of: • Decreased overall estimated intake • Excessive consumption of convenience foods, pre-prepared meals, and foods prepared away from home resulting in an inability to adhere to nutrition prescription • Uncertainty regarding appropriate foods to prepare based on nutrition prescription • Inability to purchase and transport foods to one's home

Impaired Ability to Prepare Foods/ Meals (NB-2.4)

Client History	• Conditions associated with a diagnosis or treatment, e.g., cognitive impairment, cerebral palsy, paraplegia, vision problems, rigorous therapy regimen, recent surgery

Updated: 2009 Edition

DIAGNOSIS

Poor Nutrition Quality of Life (NQOL) (NB-2.5)

Definition
Diminished patient/client perception of quality of life in response to nutrition problems and recommendations.

Etiology (Cause/Contributing Risk Factors)
Factors gathered during the nutrition assessment process that contribute to the existence or the maintenance of pathophysiological, psychosocial, situational, developmental, cultural, and/or environmental problems:

- Food and nutrition knowledge-related deficit
- Not ready for diet/lifestyle change
- Negative impact of current or previous medical nutrition therapy (MNT)
- Food or activity behavior-related difficulty
- Poor self-efficacy
- Altered body image
- Food insecurity
- Lack of social support for implementing changes

Signs/Symptoms (Defining Characteristics)
A typical cluster of subjective and objective signs and symptoms gathered during the nutrition assessment process that provide evidence that a problem exists; quantify the problem and describe its severity.

Nutrition Assessment Category	Potential Indicators of This Nutrition Diagnosis (one or more must be present)
Biochemical Data, Medical Tests and Procedures	
Anthropometric Measurements	
Nutrition-Focused Physical Findings	

Poor Nutrition Quality of Life (NQOL) (NB-2.5)

Food/Nutrition-Related History	Reports or observations of: • Unfavorable NQOL rating • Unfavorable ratings on measure of QOL, such as SF-36 (multipurpose health survey form with 36 questions) or EORTC QLQ-C30 (quality of life tool developed for patient/clients with cancer) • Food insecurity/unwillingness to use community services that are available • Frustration or dissatisfaction with MNT recommendations • Frustration over lack of control • Inaccurate or incomplete information related to MNT recommendations • Inability to change food- or activity-related behavior • Concerns about previous attempts to learn information • MNT recommendations affecting socialization • Unwillingness or disinterest in learning information
Client History	• New medical diagnosis or change in existing diagnosis or condition • Recent other lifestyle or life changes, e.g., quit smoking, initiated exercise, work change, home relocation • Lack of social and familial support • Ethnic and cultural related issues

DIAGNOSIS

Updated: 2008 Edition

Self-Feeding Difficulty (NB-2.6)

Definition
Impaired actions to place food or beverages in mouth.

Etiology (Cause/Contributing Risk Factors)
Factors gathered during the nutrition assessment process that contribute to the existence or the maintenance of pathophysiological, psychosocial, situational, developmental, cultural, and/or environmental problems:

- Physiological difficulty causing inability to physically grasp cups and utensils, support and/or control head and neck, coordinate hand movement to mouth, close lips (or any other suckling issue), bend elbow or wrist, sit with hips square and back straight
- Limited physical strength or range of motion
- Lack of or limited access to foods and/or adaptive eating devices conducive for self-feeding
- Limited vision
- Impaired cognitive ability, including learning disabilities, neurological or sensory impairment, and/or dementia
- Reluctance or avoidance of self-feeding

Signs/Symptoms (Defining Characteristics)
A typical cluster of subjective and objective signs and symptoms gathered during the nutrition assessment process that provide evidence that a problem exists; quantify the problem and describe its severity.

Nutrition Assessment Category	Potential Indicators of This Nutrition Diagnosis (one or more must be present)
Biochemical Data, Medical Tests and Procedures	
Anthropometric Measurements	• Weight loss
Nutrition-Focused Physical Findings	• Dry mucous membranes, hoarse or wet voice, tongue extrusion • Poor lip closure, drooling • Shortness of breath

Self-Feeding Difficulty (NB-2.6)

Food/Nutrition-Related History	Reports or observations of: • Being provided with foods that may not be conducive to self-feeding, e.g., peas, broth-type soups • Dropping of cups, utensils • Emotional distress, anxiety, or frustration surrounding mealtimes • Failure to recognize foods • Forgets to eat • Less than optimal use of food • Refusal to eat or chew • Dropping of food from utensil (splashing and spilling of food) on repeated attempts to feed • Lack of strength or stamina to lift utensils and/or cup • Utensil biting • Absence of recommended adaptive eating devices
Client History	• Conditions associated with a diagnosis or treatment, e.g., neurological disorders, Parkinson's, Alzheimer's, Tardive dyskinesia, multiple sclerosis, stroke, paralysis, developmental delay • Physical limitations, e.g., fractured arms, traction, contractures • Surgery requiring recumbent position • Dementia/organic brain syndrome • Dysphagia • Tremors

Updated: 2009 Edition

DIAGNOSIS

4th Edition

Intake of Unsafe Food (NB-3.1)

Definition

Intake of food and/or fluids intentionally or unintentionally contaminated with toxins, poisonous products, infectious agents, microbial agents, additives, allergens, and/or agents of bioterrorism.

Etiology (Cause/Contributing Risk Factors)

Factors gathered during the nutrition assessment process that contribute to the existence or the maintenance of pathophysiological, psychosocial, situational, developmental, cultural, and/or environmental problems:

- Food and nutrition-related knowledge deficit concerning potentially unsafe food
- Lack of knowledge about proper food/feeding, (infant and enteral formula, breastmilk*) storage, and preparation
- Exposure to contaminated water or food, e.g., community outbreak of illness documented by surveillance and/or response agency
- Mental illness, confusion, or altered awareness
- Lack of or limited access to food storage equipment/facilities, e.g., refrigerator
- Lack of or limited access to safe food supply, e.g., inadequate markets with safe, uncontaminated food

Signs/Symptoms (Defining Characteristics)

A typical cluster of subjective and objective signs and symptoms gathered during the nutrition assessment process that provide evidence that a problem exists; quantify the problem and describe its severity.

Nutrition Assessment Category	Potential Indicators of This Nutrition Diagnosis (one or more must be present)
Biochemical Data, Medical Tests and Procedures	• Positive stool culture for infectious causes, such as listeria, salmonella, hepatitis A, E. coli, cyclospora • Toxicology reports for drugs, medicinals, poisons in blood or food samples
Anthropometric Measurements	
Nutrition-Focused Physical Findings	• Evidence of dehydration, e.g., dry mucous membranes, damaged tissues • Diarrhea, cramping, bloating, fever, nausea, vomiting, vision problems, chills, dizziness, headache

If a synonym for the term "breastmilk" is helpful or needed, an approved alternate is "human milk."

Intake of Unsafe Food (NB-3.1)

Food/Nutrition-Related History	Reports or observations of: • Fish suspected to contain mercury (pregnant and lactating women) • Nonfood items (pregnant and lactating women) • Raw eggs, unpasteurized milk products, soft cheeses, undercooked meats (infants, children, immunocompromised persons, pregnant and lactating women, and elderly) • Wild plants, berries, mushrooms • Unsafely stored and prepared foods or products (enteral and infant formula, breastmilk) • Mislabeled or unlabeled foods • Verbalizes inaccurate or incomplete knowledge
Client History	• Conditions associated with a diagnosis or treatment, e.g., foodborne illness such as bacterial, viral, or parasitic infection, mental illness, dementia • Poisoning by drugs, medicinals, and biological substances • Poisoning from poisonous food stuffs and poisonous plants • Cardiac, neurologic, respiratory changes

Updated: 2013 Edition

DIAGNOSIS

4th Edition

Limited Access to Food and/or Water (NB-3.2)

Definition
Diminished ability to acquire a sufficient quantity and variety of healthful food and/or potable water based on dietary reference intake standards (e.g., Dietary Reference Intakes), national food guidelines (e.g., US Dietary Guidelines, MyPlate) or as defined in the nutrition prescription.

Etiology (Cause/Contributing Risk Factors)
Factors gathered during the nutrition assessment process that contribute to the existence or the maintenance of pathophysiological, psychosocial, situational, developmental, cultural, and/or environmental problems:

- Caregiver intentionally or unintentionally not providing access to food and/or water, e.g., unmet needs for food or eating assistance, excess of poor nutritional quality food, abuse/neglect
- Community and geographical constraints for shopping and transportation
- Food and nutrition-related knowledge deficit concerning sufficient quantity or variety of culturally appropriate healthful food and/or water
- Lack of financial resources or lack of access to financial resources to purchase a sufficient quantity or variety of culturally appropriate healthful foods and/or water
- Lack of food planning, purchasing, and preparation skills
- Limited, absent, or lack of participation in community supplemental food or other programs, e.g., food pantries, emergency kitchens, or shelters
- Failure to participate in federal food programs, e.g., WIC, National School Breakfast/Lunch Program, food stamps
- Schools lacking nutrition/wellness policies or application of policies ensuring convenient, appetizing, competitively priced culturally appropriate healthful foods at meals, snacks, and school-sponsored activities.
- Physical or psychological limitations that diminish ability to shop, e.g., walking, sight, mental/emotional health
- Limitation to food because of concerns about weight or aging

Signs/Symptoms (Defining Characteristics)
A typical cluster of subjective and objective signs and symptoms gathered during the nutrition assessment process that provide evidence that a problem exists; quantify the problem and describe its severity.

Nutrition Assessment Category	Potential Indicators of This Nutrition Diagnosis (one or more must be present)
Biochemical Data, Medical Tests and Procedures	• Indicators of macronutrient or vitamin/mineral status as indicated by biochemical findings • Evidence of dehydration, e.g., dry mucous membranes, poor skin turgor

Limited Access to Food and/or Water (NB-3.2)

Anthropometric Measurements	• Growth failure, based on reference growth standards, e.g., National Center for Health Statistics (NCHS) • Underweight: BMI < 18.5 (adults) • Unintetional weight loss: adults, of > 10% in 6 months, > 5% in 1 month; any unintentional weight loss in children • Overweight/obesity: BMI > 25 (adults), > 95 percentile (pediatrics)
Nutrition-Focused Physical Findings	• Findings consistent with vitamin/mineral deficiency • Hunger, thirst
Food/Nutrition-Related History	Reports or observations of: • Food faddism or unsupported beliefs and attitudes of parent or caregiver • Belief that aging can be slowed by dietary limitations and extreme exercise • Estimated inadequate intake of food and/or specific nutrients • Limited supply of food and/or water in home • Limited variety of foods • Lack of resources for food and/or water • Lack of transportation or other community constraints limiting availability of food and/or water • Lack of knowledge or skills on how to use food • Lack of knowledge or skills on how to apply and/or participate in food and/or water assistance programs • Behaviors consistent with food insecurity (e.g., skipping meals, buying low-cost food items, changes in eating patterns, rituals, or customs)
Client History	• Malnutrition, vitamin/mineral deficiency • Illness or physical disability • Conditions associated with a diagnosis or treatment, e.g., mental illness, dementia • Lack of suitable support systems

DIAGNOSIS

Updated: 2013 Edition

Limited Access to Nutrition-Related Supplies (NB-3.3)

Definition
Diminished ability to acquire nutrition-related supplies based on identified needs.

Etiology (Cause/Contributing Risk Factors)
Factors gathered during the nutrition assessment process that contribute to the existence or the maintenance of pathophysiological, psychosocial, situational, developmental, cultural, and/or environmental problems:

- Caregiver intentionally or unintentionally not providing access to nutrition-related supplies, e.g., unmet needs, abuse/neglect
- Community and geographical constraints for shopping and transportation to obtain nutrition-related supplies
- Food and nutrition-related knowledge deficit concerning nutrition-related supplies
- Lack of financial resources or lack of access to financial resources to purchase nutrition-related supplies
- Limited, absent, or failure to participate in community or other programs that provide access to nutrition-related supplies
- Physical or psychological limitations that diminish ability to shop, e.g., walking, sight, mental/emotional health

Signs/Symptoms (Defining Characteristics)
A typical cluster of subjective and objective signs and symptoms gathered during the nutrition assessment process that provide evidence that a problem exists; quantify the problem and describe its severity.

Nutrition Assessment Category	Potential Indicators of This Nutrition Diagnosis (one or more must be present)
Biochemical Data, Medical Tests and Procedures	• Abnormal biochemical findings consistent with vitamin/mineral deficiency
Anthropometric Measurements	• Growth failure, based on reference growth standards, e.g. National Center for Health Statistics (NCHS) • Underweight: BMI <18.5 (adults) • Unintentional weight loss: adults, of > 10% in 6 months, > 5% in 1 month; any unintentional weight loss in children
Nutrition-Focused Physical Findings	• Findings consistent with vitamin/mineral deficiency • Hunger, thirst • Evidence of dehydration, e.g., dry mucous membranes, poor skin turgor

DIAGNOSIS

Limited Access to Nutrition-Related Supplies (NB-3.3)

Food/Nutrition-Related History	Reports or observations of: • Food faddism or unsupported beliefs and attitudes of parent or caregiver • Limited supply of nutrition-related supplies (e.g., glucose testing strips, meter, assistive eating devices, assistive cooking devices) in home • Transportation or other community constraints limiting availability of nutrition-related supplies • Lack of knowledge or skills on how to use nutrition-related supplies • Lack of knowledge or skills on how to apply and/or participate in nutrition-related supply assistance programs
Client History	• Malnutrition, vitamin/mineral deficiency • Illness or physical disability • Conditions associated with a diagnosis or treatment, e.g., mental illness, dementia • Lack of suitable support systems • Resource constraints for obtaining nutrition-related supplies

Created: 2011 Edition

DIAGNOSIS

No Nutrition Diagnosis At This Time (NO-1.1)

Definition
Absence of a current nutrition problem warranting a nutrition intervention. This determination results from a nutrition assessment.

> *Note: This nutrition diagnositic term is not appropriate if additional information for the nutrition assessment is needed or pending.*

Etiology (Cause/Contributing Risk Factors)
Factors gathered during the nutrition assessment process that contribute to the existence or the maintenance of pathophysiological, psychosocial, situational, developmental, cultural, and/or environmental problems:

- Not applicable

Signs/Symptoms (Defining Characteristics)
A typical cluster of subjective and objective signs and symptoms gathered during the nutrition assessment process that provide evidence that a problem exists; quantify the problem and describe its severity.

Nutrition Assessment Category	Potential Indicators of This Nutrition Diagnosis (one or more must be present)
Biochemical Data, Medical Tests and Procedures	Not applicable
Anthropometric Measurements	Not applicable
Nutrition-Focused Physical Findings	Not applicable
Food/Nutrition-Related History	Not applicable
Client History	• Conditions associated with a diagnosis or treatment, e.g., palliative/end-of-life care

Created: 2013 Edition

NCP Step 3: Nutrition Intervention

What is the purpose of a nutrition intervention? The purpose is to resolve or improve the identified nutrition problem by planning and implementing appropriate nutrition interventions that are tailored to the patient/client's* needs.

How does a food and nutrition professional determine a nutrition intervention? The selection of nutrition interventions is driven by the nutrition diagnosis and its etiology. Nutrition intervention strategies are purposefully selected to change nutritional intake, nutrition-related knowledge or behavior, environmental conditions, or access to supportive care and services. Nutrition intervention goals provide the basis for monitoring progress and measuring outcomes.

How are the nutrition intervention strategies organized? In four categories:

Food and/or Nutrient Delivery—*Individualized approach for food/nutrient provision*

Nutrition Education—*A formal process to instruct or train a patient/client in a skill or to impart knowledge to help patients/clients voluntarily manage or modify food, nutrition and physical activity choices and behavior to maintain or improve health*

Nutrition Counseling—*A supportive process, characterized by a collaborative counselor-patient relationship, to establish food, nutrition and physical activity priorities, goals, and individualized action plans that acknowledge and foster responsibility for self-care to treat an existing condition and promote health*

Coordination of Nutrition Care—*Consultation with, referral to, or coordination of nutrition care with other health care providers, institutions, or agencies that can assist in treating or managing nutrition-related problems*

What does nutrition intervention involve? Nutrition intervention entails two distinct and interrelated components—planning and implementing. Planning the nutrition intervention involves (a) prioritizing nutrition diagnoses, (b) consulting the Academy's Evidence-Based Nutrition Practice Guidelines and other practice guidelines, (c) determining patient-focused expected outcomes for each nutrition diagnosis, (d) conferring with patient/client/caregivers, (e) defining a nutrition intervention plan and strategies, (f) defining time and frequency of care, and (g) identifying resources needed. Implementation is the action phase and involves (a) communication of the nutrition care plan and (b) carrying out the plan.

INTERVENTION

*Patient/client refers to individuals, groups, populations, family members, and/or caregivers.

Critical thinking during this step...
- Setting goals and prioritizing
- Defining the nutrition prescription or basic plan
- Making interdisciplinary connections
- Initiating behavioral and other nutrition interventions
- Matching nutrition intervention strategies with patient/client's needs, nutrition diagnosis, and values
- Choosing from among alternatives to determine a course of action
- Specifying the time and frequency of care

Are food and nutrition professionals limited to the defined nutrition intervention terms? Nutrition intervention terminology includes commonly used strategies and emphasizes the application of evidence-based strategies matched to appropriate circumstances. Evaluation of the nutrition intervention terminology is ongoing and will guide future modifications. Food and nutrition professionals can propose additions or revisions using the Procedure for Nutrition Controlled Vocabulary/ Terminology Maintenance/Review available from the Academy.

Detailed information about this step can be found in the Academy of Nutrition and Dietetics' International Dietetics and Nutrition Terminology (IDNT) Reference Manual: Standardized Language for the Nutrition Care Process, Fourth Edition.

Nutrition Intervention Terminology

Each term has an Academy unique identifier, a five-digit number (e.g., 99999) following the alpha-numeric IDNT code. Neither should be visible in nutrition documentation. The Academy unique identifier is for data tracking purposes in electronic records.

Nutrition Prescription   NP-1.1   10794

The patient/client's individualized recommended dietary intake of energy and/or selected foods or nutrients based on current reference standards and dietary guidelines and the patient/client's health condition and nutrition diagnosis (*specify*).

_____

_____

_____

FOOD AND/OR NUTRIENT DELIVERY   ND

Individualized approach for food /nutrient provision.

Meals and Snacks (1)

Regular eating episode (meal); food served between regular meals (snack).

❏ General/healthful diet	ND-1.1	10489
❏ Composition of meals/snacks	ND-1.2	
❏ Texture-modified diet (1)		10829
❏ Energy-modified diet (2)		10830
❏ Protein-modified diet (3)		10831
❏ Carbohydrate-modified diet (4)		10832
❏ Fat-modified diet (5)		10833
❏ Fiber-modified diet (6)		10834
❏ Fluid-modified diet (7)		10835
❏ Diets modified for specific foods or ingredients (8)		10836
❏ Vitamin-modified diet (9)		10837
❏ Mineral-modified diet (10)		10838
❏ Schedule of food/fluids	ND-1.3	10815
❏ Specific foods/beverages or groups	ND-1.4	10492
❏ Other	ND-1.5	10493
(*specify*) _____		

Enteral and Parenteral Nutrition (2)

Nutrition provided through the GI tract via tube, catheter, or stoma (enteral) or intravenously (centrally or peripherally) (parenteral).

Enteral Nutrition (2.1)

Nutrition provided through the GI tract.

❏ Composition	ND-2.1.1	10503
❏ Concentration	ND-2.1.2	10502
❏ Rate	ND-2.1.3	10500
❏ Volume	ND-2.1.4	10501
❏ Schedule	ND-2.1.5	10504
❏ Route	ND-2.1.6	10792
❏ Insert enteral feeding tube	ND-2.1.7	10497
❏ Site care	ND-2.1.8	10498
❏ Feeding tube flush	ND-2.1.9	10499

Parenteral Nutrition/IV Fluids (2.2)

Nutrition and fluids provided intravenously.

❏ Composition	ND-2.2.1	10511
❏ Concentration	ND-2.2.2	10510
❏ Rate	ND-2.2.3	10509
❏ Schedule	ND-2.2.4	10512
❏ Route	ND-2.2.5	10793
❏ Site care	ND-2.2.6	10507
❏ IV fluids	ND-2.2.7	10508

Supplements (3)

Medical Food Supplements (3.1)

Commercial or prepared foods or beverages that supplement energy, protein, carbohydrate, fiber, fat intake.

❏ Commercial beverage	ND-3.1.1	10515
❏ Commercial food	ND-3.1.2	10516
❏ Modified beverage	ND-3.1.3	10517
❏ Modified food	ND-3.1.4	10518
❏ Purpose	ND-3.1.5	10519
(*specify*) _____		

Vitamin and Mineral Supplements (3.2)

Supplemental vitamins or minerals.

❏ Multivitamin/mineral	ND-3.2.1	10521
❏ Multi-trace elements	ND-3.2.2	10522
❏ Vitamin	ND-3.2.3	
❏ A (1)		10524
❏ C (2)		10525
❏ D (3)		10526
❏ E (4)		10527
❏ K (5)		10528
❏ Thiamin (6)		10529
❏ Riboflavin (7)		10530
❏ Niacin (8)		10531
❏ Folate (9)		10532
❏ B6 (10)		10533
❏ B12 (11)		10534
❏ Pantothenic acid (12)		10535
❏ Biotin (13)		10536

INTERVENTION

□ Mineral	ND-3.2.4	
□ Calcium (1)		10539
□ Chloride (2)		10540
□ Iron (3)		10541
□ Magnesium (4)		10542
□ Potassium (5)		10543
□ Phosphorus (6)		10544
□ Sodium (7)		10545
□ Zinc (8)		10546
□ Sulfate (9)		10547
□ Fluoride (10)		10548
□ Copper (11)		10549
□ Iodine (12)		10550
□ Selenium (13)		10551
□ Manganese (14)		10552
□ Chromium (15)		10553
□ Molybdenum (16)		10554
□ Boron (17)		10555
□ Cobalt (18)		10556

Bioactive Substance Management (3.3)
Addition or change in provision of bioactive substances.

□ Plant stanol esters	ND-3.3.1	10559
□ Plant sterol esters	ND-3.3.2	10816
□ Soy protein	ND-3.3.3	10561
□ Psyllium	ND-3.3.4	10817
□ β-glucan	ND-3.3.5	10563
□ Food additives (*specify*)	ND-3.3.6	10564
□ Alcohol	ND-3.3.7	10565
□ Caffeine	ND-3.3.8	10566
□ Other (*specify*)	ND-3.3.9	10567

Feeding Assistance (4)
Accommodation or assistance in eating.

□ Adaptive eating device	ND-4.1	10808
□ Feeding position	ND-4.2	10570
□ Meal set-up	ND-4.3	10571
□ Mouth care	ND-4.4	10572
□ Menu selection assistance	ND-4.5	10809
□ Other	ND-4.6	10573
(*specify*) _____		

Feeding Environment (5)
Adjustment of the factors where food is served that impact food consumption.

□ Lighting	ND-5.1	10575
□ Odors	ND-5.2	10576
□ Distractions	ND-5.3	10577
□ Table height	ND-5.4	10578
□ Table service	ND-5.5	10849
□ Room temperature	ND-5.6	10580
□ Meal service	ND-5.7	10810
□ Meal location	ND-5.8	10811
□ Other	ND-5.9	10581
(*specify*) _____		

Nutrition-Related Medication Management (6)
Modification of a medication or complementary/ alternative medicine to optimize patient/client nutritional or health status.

□ Prescription medications	ND-6.1	10839
□ OTC medication	ND-6.2	10584
□ Nutrition-related complementary/alternative medicine	ND-6.3	10799

NUTRITION EDUCATION   E
Formal process to instruct or train patients/clients in a skill or to impart knowledge to help patients/ clients voluntarily manage or modify food, nutrition and physical activity choices and behavior to maintain or improve health.

Nutrition Education–Content (1)
Instruction or training intended to lead to nutrition-related knowledge.

□ Purpose of the nutrition education	E-1.1	10588
□ Priority modifications	E-1.2	10589
□ Survival information	E-1.3	10590
□ Nutrition relationship to health/disease	E-1.4	10591
□ Recommended modifications	E-1.5	10592
□ Other or related topics	E-1.6	10593
□ Other	E-1.7	10594
(*specify*) _____		

Nutrition Education–Application (2)
Instruction or training leading to nutrition-related result interpretation or skills.

□ Result interpretation	E-2.1	10596
□ Skill development	E-2.2	10597
□ Other	E-2.3	10598
(*specify*) _____		

NUTRITION COUNSELING   C
A supportive process, characterized by a collaborative counselor–patient/client relationship to establish food, nutrition and physical activity priorities, goals, and individualized action plans that acknowledge and foster responsibility for self-care to treat an existing condition and promote health.

Theoretical Basis/Approach (1)
The theories or models used to design and implement an intervention.

□ Cognitive-Behavioral Theory	C-1.1	10601
□ Health Belief Model	C-1.2	10602
□ Social Learning Theory	C-1.3	10603
□ Transtheoretical Model/ Stages of Change	C-1.4	10604
□ Other	C-1.5	10605
(*specify*) _____		

Strategies (2)

Selectively applied evidence-based methods or plans of action designed to achieve a particular goal.

- ❏ Motivational interviewing C-2.1   10607
- ❏ Goal setting   C-2.2   10608
- ❏ Self-monitoring   C-2.3   10609
- ❏ Problem solving   C-2.4   10610
- ❏ Social support   C-2.5   10611
- ❏ Stress management   C-2.6   10612
- ❏ Stimulus control   C-2.7   10613
- ❏ Cognitive restructuring   C-2.8   10614
- ❏ Relapse prevention   C-2.9   10615
- ❏ Rewards/contingency management   C-2.10   10616
- ❏ Other   C-2.11   10617
  (*specify*) _____

COORDINATION OF NUTRITION CARE   RC

Consultation with, referral to, or coordination of nutrition care with other providers, institutions, or agencies that can assist in treating or managing nutrition-related problems.

Collaboration and Referral of Nutrition Care (1)

Facilitating services with other professionals, institutions, or agencies during nutrition care.

- ❏ Team meeting   RC-1.1   10620
- ❏ Referral to RD with different expertise   RC-1.2   10621
- ❏ Collaboration with other nutrition professionals   RC-1.3   10622
- ❏ Collaboration with other providers   RC-1.4   10623
- ❏ Referral to other providers   RC-1.5   10624
- ❏ Referral to community agencies/programs (*specify*)   RC-1.6   10625 _____

Discharge and Transfer of Nutrition Care to New Setting or Provider (2)

Discharge planning and transfer of nutrition care from one level or location of care to another.

- ❏ Discharge and transfer to other providers   RC-2.1   10813
- ❏ Discharge and transfer to community agencies/programs   RC-2.2   10814
- ❏ Discharge and transfer to another nutrition professional   RC-2.3   10627

INTERVENTION

Nutrition Prescription (NP-1.1)

Definition

The patient/client's recommended dietary intake of energy and/or selected foods or nutrients based on current reference standards and dietary guidelines and the patient/client's health condition and nutrition diagnosis

Purpose

To communicate the nutrition professional's diet/nutrition recommendation based on a nutrition assessment

Indicators

- Recommended regular diet
- Recommended modified diet
  - Recommended energy/nutrient modification
    - Calorie modification (specify, e.g., calories/day, calories/kg/day)
    - Recommended carbohydrate modification
      - Carbohydrate controlled diet (specify, e.g., distribution)
      - Amount (specify, e.g., grams/day, grams/kg/min, percent of calories)
      - Other (specify, e.g., no concentrated sweets)
    - Recommended protein level (specify, e.g., grams/day, grams/kg/day, percent of calories)
    - Recommended fat level (specify, e.g., grams/day, grams/kg/day, percent of calories)
      - Fat restricted diet (specify, e.g., grams/day)
      - Therapeutic lifestyle change diet
      - Recommended saturated fat level (specify, e.g., grams/day, percent of calories)
      - Recommended unsaturated fat level (specify, e.g., grams/day, percent of calories)
      - Recommended cholesterol intake (specify, e.g., mg/day)
    - Recommended vitamin intake
      - Vitamin A (specify form, µg or RE, frequency)
      - Vitamin C (mg/ day, frequency)
      - Vitamin D (specify form, µg or IU, frequency)
      - Vitamin E (specify form, mg or IU, frequency)
      - Vitamin K (µg, frequency)
      - Thiamin (mg, frequency)
      - Riboflavin (mg, frequency)
      - Niacin (specify form, mg, frequency)
      - Vitamin B6 (specify form, mg, frequency)
      - Folate (specify form, µg, frequency)
      - Vitamin B12 (µg, frequency)
      - Pantothenic acid (mg, frequency)
      - Biotin (µg, frequency)
      - Multivitamin (yes/no, specify dose, frequency)

INTERVENTION

Nutrition Prescription (NP-1.1)

- Recommended mineral intake
  - Calcium (specify form, mg, frequency)
  - Copper (μg or mg, frequency)
  - Fluoride (mg, frequency)
  - Iodine (μg, frequency)
  - Iron (specify form, mg, frequency)
  - Magnesium (mg, frequency)
  - Phosphorus (mg, frequency)
  - Sulfate (g or mmol, frequency)
  - Manganese (mg, frequency)
  - Molybdenum (μg, frequency)
  - Boron (mg, frequency)
  - Cobalt (μg, frequency)
  - Selenium (specify form, μg, frequency)
  - Zinc (mg, frequency)
  - Potassium (specify form, g or mg, frequency)
  - Chloride (mg, frequency)
  - Chromium (specify form, μg, frequency)
  - Multi-mineral (yes/no, specify dose, frequency)
  - Multi-trace element (yes/no, specify dose, frequency)
- Recommended fluid level (specify, e.g., oz or mL/day, mL/kg/day, mL per calories/kcal/kJ expended, mL/m^2/day, mL output)
- Recommended fiber level (specify, e.g., type, grams/day, grams/1,000 calories/kcal/kJ per day)
- Recommended level of bioactive substances (specify, e.g., substance, amount)
- Recommended enteral nutrition order (specify, e.g., formula, rate/schedule)
  - Tube feeding modulars (specify, e.g., carbohydrate, protein, fat, fiber)
- Recommended parenteral nutrition order (specify, e.g., solution, rate, access)
- Recommended liquid diet
  - Clear liquid
  - Full liquid
- Recommended texture modification (specify, e.g., mechanical soft, puree)
- Recommended liquid consistency modification (specify, e.g., thin, nectar, honey, pudding)
- Recommended food intake
  - Grain group intake (specify, e.g., servings, exchanges, amounts)
  - Fruit and vegetable intake (specify, e.g., servings, exchanges, amounts)
  - Meat, poultry, fish, eggs, beans, nut intake (specify, e.g., servings, exchanges, amounts)
  - Milk and milk product intake (specify, e.g., servings, exchanges, amounts)
  - Fat foods (specify, e.g., type, servings, exchanges, amounts

Note: The nutrition prescription can be used as a comparative standard for nutrition assessment and nutrition monitoring and evaluation.

INTERVENTION

Meals and Snacks (ND-1)

Definition
Meals are defined as regular eating episodes that may include a variety of foods consisting of grains and/or starches, meat and/or meat alternatives, fruits and vegetables, and milk or milk products. A snack is defined as food served between regular meals.

Details of Intervention
A typical intervention might be further described with the following details. RDs/food and nutrition professionals recommend, implement, or order nutrition interventions and the action(s) may be to initiate, modify or discontinue a nutrition intervention(s):

- General/healthful diet
- Composition of meals/snacks
  - Texture-modified diet
  - Energy-modified diet
  - Protein-modified diet
  - Carbohydrate-modified diet
  - Fat-modified diet
  - Fiber-modified diet
  - Fluid-modified diet
  - Diets modified for specific foods or ingredients
  - Vitamin-modified diet
  - Mineral-modified diet
- Schedule of food/fluids (e.g., timing of foods/fluids, number of meals)
- Specific food/beverages or groups
- Other, specify

See reference manual for list of nutrition diagnoses, etiologies and signs and symptoms that often are associated with this intervention.

Other considerations (e.g., patient/client negotiation, patient/client needs and desires, and readiness to change)

- Compliance skills and abilities
- Economic concerns with purchasing special food items
- Willingness/ability to change behavior to comply with diet
- Availability/access to a qualified practitioner for follow-up and monitoring

Updated: 2013 Edition

INTERVENTION

Enteral Nutrition (ND-2.1)

Definition
Nutrition provided through the gastrointestinal (GI) tract via tube, catheter, or stoma that delivers nutrients distal to the oral cavity

Details of Intervention
A typical intervention might be further described with the following details. RDs/food and nutrition professionals recommend, implement, or order nutrition interventions and the action(s) may be to initiate, modify or discontinue a nutrition intervention(s):

- Composition: formula name or description, special additives including supplemental fat, carbohydrate, or protein, fiber or other (specify)
- Concentration (e.g., calories/kcal/kJ per mL)
- Rate (e.g., mL/hour)
- Volume (e.g., mL/day, mL/feeding)
- Schedule (e.g., number of hours per 24 hours, continuous, intermittent, bolus)
- Route (e.g., nasoentric, oroenteric, percutaneous, or surgical access with gastric, duodenal or jejunal placement)
- Insert enteral feeding tube
- Site care (e.g., change dressings and provide enteral feeding tube site care)
- Feeding tube flush (e.g., type, volume mL/flush, frequency)

Note:Related nutrition interventions, e.g., checking gastric residual volume or elevating the head of the bed are documented using Coordination of Nutrition Care

See reference manual for list of nutrition diagnoses, etiologies and signs and symptoms that often are associated with this intervention.

Other considerations (e.g., patient/client negotiation, patient/client needs and desires, and readiness to change)

- End-of-life issues, ethical considerations, patient/client rights and family/caregiver issues
- Other nutrient intake (oral, parenteral, or enteral nutrition)
- Enteral formulary composition and product availability
- Availability/access to a qualified practitioner for follow-up and monitoring
- Economic constraints that limit availability of food/enteral products

Updated: 2013 Edition

Parenteral Nutrition/IV Fluids (ND-2.2)

Definition

Administration of nutrients and fluids intravenously, centrally (delivered into a large-diameter vein, usually the superior vena cava adjacent to the right atrium) or peripherally (delivered into a peripheral vein, usually of the hand or forearm).

Details of Intervention

A typical intervention might be further described with the following details: RDs/food and nutrition professionals recommend, implement, or order nutrition interventions and the action(s) may be to initiate, modify or discontinue a nutrition intervention(s):

- Composition (formula or description)
- Concentration (e.g., percent, grams of solute per mL)
- Rate (e.g., mL/hour)
- Schedule (e.g., hours, timing, taper schedule)
- Route (e.g., peripheral, central, and/or type of catheter)
- Site care (e.g., change dressings and provide line care for parenteral access)
- IV fluids (e.g., type; amount mL/day, mL/hr, mL with medications)

See reference manual for list of nutrition diagnoses, etiologies and signs and symptoms that often are associated with this intervention.

Other considerations (e.g., patient/client negotiation, patient/client needs and desires, and readiness to change)

- End-of-life issues, ethical considerations, patient/client rights and family/ caregiver issues
- Other nutrient intake (oral, parenteral, or enteral nutrition)
- Parenteral formulary composition and product availability
- Availability/access to a qualified practitioner for follow-up and monitoring
- Economic constraints that limit availability of parenteral products

INTERVENTION

Updated: 2013 Edition

Medical Food Supplements (ND-3.1)

Definition

Commercial or prepared foods or beverages intended to supplement energy, protein, carbohydrate, fiber, and/or fat intake that may also contribute to vitamin and mineral intake.

Details of Intervention

A typical intervention might be further described with the following details: RDs/food and nutrition professionals recommend, implement, or order nutrition interventions and the action(s) may be to initiate, modify or discontinue a nutrition intervention(s):

- Commercial (prepackaged) beverage
- Commercial (prepackaged) food
- Modified (prepared) beverage
- Modified (prepared) food
- Purpose (e.g., to supplement energy, protein, carbohydrate, fiber, and/or fat intake)

See reference manual for list of nutrition diagnoses, etiologies and signs and symptom that often are associated with this intervention.

Other considerations (e.g., patient/client negotiation, patient/client needs and desires, and readiness to change)

- Appetite sufficient to take medical food supplements
- System constraints that prevent meeting the client's preferences for specific flavors, textures, foods, and the timing of feedings
- Availability of feeding assistance
- Economic concerns and product/food availability

Updated: 2013 Edition

Vitamin and Mineral Supplements (ND-3.2)

Definition

A product that is intended to supplement vitamin or mineral intake.

Details of Intervention

A typical intervention might be further described with the following details:
RDs/food and nutrition professionals recommend, implement, or order nutrition interventions and the action(s) may be to initiate, modify or discontinue a nutrition intervention(s):

- Vitamin supplement:
    - Vitamin A (specify form, μg or RE, frequency)
    - Vitamin C (mg/ day, frequency)
    - Vitamin D (specify form, μg or IU, frequency)
    - Vitamin E (specify form, mg or IU, frequency)
    - Vitamin K (μg, frequency)
    - Thiamin (mg, frequency)
    - Riboflavin (mg, frequency)
    - Multivitamin (yes/no, specify dose, frequency)
    - Niacin (specify form, mg, frequency)
    - Vitamin B6 (specify form, mg, frequency)
    - Folate (specify form, μg, frequency)
    - Vitamin B12 (μg, frequency)
    - Pantothenic acid (mg, frequency)
    - Biotin (μg, frequency)

- Mineral supplement:
    - Calcium (specify form, mg, frequency)
    - Copper (μg or mg, frequency)
    - Fluoride (mg, frequency)
    - Iodine (μg, frequency)
    - Iron (specify form, mg, frequency)
    - Magnesium (mg, frequency)
    - Phosphorus (mg, frequency)
    - Sulfate (g or mmol, frequency)
    - Manganese (mg, frequency)
    - Multi-mineral (yes/no, specify dose, frequency)
    - Molybdenum (μg, frequency)
    - Boron (mg, frequency)
    - Cobalt (μg, frequency)
    - Selenium (specify form, μg, frequency)
    - Zinc (mg, frequency)
    - Potassium (specify form, g or mg, frequency)
    - Sodium (mg or g, frequency)
    - Chloride (mg, frequency)
    - Chromium (specify form, μg, frequency)
    - Multi-trace element (yes/no, specify dose, frequency)

See reference manual for list of nutrition diagnoses, etiologies and signs and symptoms that often are associated with this intervention.

Other considerations (e.g., patient/client negotiation, patient/client needs and desires, and readiness to change)

- Emerging scientific evidence to support the use of vitamin and mineral supplements in specific populations
- Availability of a qualified practitioner with additional education/training in the use of vitamin and mineral supplements in practice
- Economic considerations and product availability

Updated: 2013 Edition

INTERVENTION

Bioactive Substance Management (ND-3.3)

Definition

Addition or change in provision of bioactive substances (e.g., plant stanol and sterol esters, psyllium, food additives, other bioactive substances).

Details of Intervention

A typical intervention might be further described with the following details. RDs/food and nutrition professionals recommend, implement, or order nutrition interventions and the action(s) may be to initiate, modify or discontinue a nutrition intervention(s):

- Plant stanol esters (specify g, form, frequency)
- Plant sterol esters (specify g, form, frequency)
- Soy protein (specify g, form, frequency)
- Psyllium (specify g, form, frequency)
- β-glucan (specify g, form, frequency)
- Food additives (those thought to have an impact on a patient/client's health) (specify, e.g., amount, form, frequency)
- Alcohol (specify, oz/mL, form, frequency)
- Caffeine (specify, e.g., mg, oz/mL, form, frequency)
- Other substance (for which there is evidence of bioactivity) (specify, e.g., amount, form, freqency)

See reference manual for list of nutrition diagnoses, etiologies and signs and symptom that often are associated with this intervention.

Other considerations (e.g., patient/client negotiation, patient/client needs and desires, and readiness to change)

- Emerging scientific evidence to support the use of bioactive supplements in specific populations
- Availability of a qualified practitioner with additional education/training in the use of bioactive supplements in practice

Updated: 2011 Edition

Feeding Assistance (ND-4)

efinition

ccommodation or assistance designed to restore the patient/client's ability to
t independently, support adequate nutrient intake, and reduce the incidence of
planned weight loss and dehydration.

etails of Intervention

typical intervention might be further described with the following details.
Ds/food and nutrition professionals recommend, implement, or order nutrition
terventions and the action(s) may be to initiate, modify or discontinue a nutrition
tervention(s):

- Adaptive eating devices (equipment or utensils) (e.g., specify)
- Feeding position (e.g, specify patient/client position in relationship to eating
  or degree angle for enteral feeding)
- Meal set-up (e.g., specify actions to make food accessible for consumption)
- Mouth care (e.g. specify treatment to promote oral health and hygiene)
- Menu selection assistance (yes/no)
- Other (specify)

*e reference manual for list of nutrition diagnoses, etiologies and signs and symptoms
at often are associated with this intervention.*

ther considerations (e.g., patient/client negotiation, patient/client needs and
sires, and readiness to change)

- Acceptance of feeding assistance/feeding devices
- Poor environment to foster adequate intake
- Lack of individual to provide assistance at meal time
- Lack of training in methods of feeding assistance
- Lack of available physical therapy, occupational therapy, or speech therapy
  evaluations
- Ability to understand the reasoning behind the recommendations and then
  want to make personal changes

INTERVENTION

dated: 2013 Edition

Feeding Environment (ND-5)

Definition
Adjustment of the physical environment, temperature, convenience, and attractiveness of the location where food is served that impacts food consumption.

Details of Intervention
A typical intervention might be further described with the following details. RDs/food and nutrition professionals recommend, implement, or order nutrition interventions and the action(s) may be to initiate, modify or discontinue a nutrition intervention(s):

- Lighting (e.g., specify)
- Odors (e.g., specify, minimize or enhance)
- Distractions (e.g., specify, minimize)
- Table height (specify)
- Table service (e.g., plates, napkins)
- Room temperature
- Meal service (type of service, e.g., service at table, buffet)
- Meal location (specify)
- Other

See reference manual for list of nutrition diagnoses, etiologies and signs and symptom that often are associated with this intervention.

Other considerations (e.g., patient/client negotiation, patient/client needs and desires, and readiness to change)

- Resources available to improve/modify the feeding environment

Updated: 2013 Edition

INTERVENTION

Nutrition-Related Medication Management (ND-6)

Definition

Modification of a drug or nutrition-related complementary/alternative medicine to optimize patient/client nutritional or health status.

Details of Intervention

A typical intervention might be further described with the following details. RDs/food and nutrition professionals recommend, implement, or order nutrition interventions and the action(s) may be to initiate, modify or discontinue a nutrition intervention(s):

- Prescription medication (e.g., insulin, appetite stimulants, digestive enzymes) dose, form, schedule, route
- Over-the-counter (OTC) medication (e.g., antacids, aspirin, laxatives) dose, form, schedule, route
- Nutrition-related complementary/alternative medicine (e.g., peppermint oil, probiotics), dose, form, schedule, route

See reference manual for list of nutrition diagnoses, etiologies and signs and symptoms that often are associated with this intervention.

Other considerations (e.g., patient/client negotiation, patient/client needs and desires, and readiness to change)

- Availability/access to a clinical pharmacist
- Availability of a qualified practitioner with appropriate pharmacology training and/or education

Updated: 2013 Edition

INTERVENTION

Nutrition Education–Content (E-1)

Definition
Instruction or training intended to lead to nutrition-related knowledge.

> *Note: This reference sheet only refers to patient/client nutrition education. Please use Nutrition Counseling (C) for documentation of the Theoretical Basis/Approach (C-1) and Strategies (C-2) used for patient/client behavior change.*

Details of Intervention
A typical intervention might be further described with the following details. RDs/food and nutrition professionals recommend, implement, or order nutrition interventions and the action(s) may be to initiate, modify or discontinue a nutrition intervention(s):

- Purpose (e.g., prevention, disease management) of the nutrition education
- Priority modifications (e.g., issue of most concern to patient/client's health and well-being)
- Survival information (minimum necessary nutrition modifications until patient/client can return for more nutrition education)
- Nutrition and physical activity relationship to health/disease
- Recommended modifications (e.g., explain multiple nutrition prescription recommendations)
- Other or related topics (e.g., saturated and trans fatty acid intake versus total fat intake, menu planning, food purchasing, physical activity recommendations)
- Other, specify

See reference manual for list of nutrition diagnoses, etiologies and signs and symptoms that often are associated with this intervention.

Other considerations (e.g., patient/client negotiation, patient/client needs and desires, and readiness to change)

- Met with several providers in one day and is unable or unwilling to receive more nutrition education at this time
- Profile reflects complicated situation warranting additional education/instruction
- Being discharged from the hospital
- Caregiver unavailable at time of nutrition education
- Baseline knowledge
- Learning style
- Other education and learning needs, e.g., new medication or other treatment administration

Updated: 2013 Edition

INTERVENTION

Nutrition Education–Application (E-2)

efinition

struction or training intended to lead to nutrition-related result interpretation or ills.

> *Note: This reference sheet only refers to patient/client nutrition education. Please use Nutrition Counseling (C) for documentation of the Theoretical Basis/Approach (C-1) and Strategies (C-2) used for patient/client behavior change.*

etails of Intervention

typical intervention might be further described with the following details. Ds/food and nutrition professionals recommend, implement, or order nutrition terventions and the action(s) may be to initiate, modify or discontinue a nutrition tervention(s):

- Result interpretation (e.g., engage in training on medical or other results to coincide with nutrition prescription, such as, distribution of carbohydrates throughout the day based on blood glucose monitoring results, heart rate during physical activity
- Skill development, e.g., glucometer use, home tube feeding and feeding pump training, cooking skills/preparation, physical activity equipment
- Other, specify

e reference manual for list of nutrition diagnoses, etiologies and signs and symptoms at often are associated with this intervention.

ther considerations (e.g., patient/client negotiation, patient/client needs and sires, and readiness to change)

- Profile reflects complicated situation warranting additional education/instruction
- Increased capacity and willingness to learn information
- Quality of life may be enhanced with in-depth nutrition education and understanding
- Baseline knowledge
- Lifestyle factors
- Education approaches that enhance knowledge/skill transfer

INTERVENTION

dated: 2013 Edition

Theoretical Basis/Approach (C-1)

Definition

The theories or models used to design and implement an intervention. Theories and theoretical models consist of principles, constructs, and variables, which offer systematic explanations of the human behavior change process. Behavior change theories and models provide a research-based rationale for designing and tailoring nutrition interventions to achieve the desired effect. A theoretical framework for curriculum and treatment protocols, it guides determination of: (1) what information patients/clients need at different points in the behavior change process, (2) what tool and strategies may be best applied to facilitate behavior change, and (3) outcome measures to assess effectiveness in interventions or components of interventions.

Application Guidance

One or more of the following theories or theoretical models may influence a practitioner's counseling style or approach. Practitioners are asked to identify those theories (C-1) that most influence the intervention being documented. An intervention might also incorporate tools and strategies derived from a variety of behavior change theories and models. The practitioner is also asked to indicate which strategies (C-2) they used in a particular intervention session.

Details of Intervention

A typical intervention might be further described with the following details. RDs/foo and nutrition professionals recommend, implement, or order nutrition interventions and the action(s) may be to initiate, modify or discontinue a nutrition intervention(s)

The following theories and models have proven valuable in providing a theoretical framework for evidence-based individual and interpersonal level nutrition interven tions. Other theories may be useful for community level interventions (e.g., Community Organization, Diffusion of Innovations, Communication Theory).

- Cognitive-Behavioral Theory
- Health Belief Model
- Social Learning Theory
- Transtheoretical Model/Stages of Change

Additional information regarding each of the above theories and models can be found within this reference sheet.

See reference manual for list of nutrition diagnoses, etiologies and signs and sympto *that often are associated with this intervention.*

Other considerations (e.g., patient/client negotiation, patient/client needs and desires, and readiness to change)

- Lifestyle factors
- Language barrier
- Educational level
- Culture
- Socioeconomic status

Theoretical Basis/Approach (C-1)

Cognitive-Behavioral Theory

escription

ognitive-Behavioral Theory (CBT) is based on the assumption that all behavior
learned and is directly related to internal factors (e.g., thoughts and thinking
tterns) and external factors (e.g., environmental stimulus and reinforcement) that
e related to the problem behaviors. Application involves use of both cognitive and
havioral change strategies to effect behavior change.

plication for Counseling Interventions

3T, derived from an educational model, is based on the assumption that most
notional and behavioral reactions are learned and can be unlearned. The goal of
3T is to facilitate client identification of cognitions and behaviors that lead to less-
an-optimal eating or exercise habits and replace these with more rational thoughts
d actions.

e process is:

- Goal directed
- Process oriented
- Facilitated through a variety of problem-solving tools

havioral and cognitive techniques to modify eating and exercise habits are taught
r continuous application by the patient/client. Practitioners implement Cognitive-
havioral Theory by partnering with clients to study their current environment to:

- • Identify determinants or antecedents to behavior that contribute to less
  than optimal eating/exercise
- Identify resultant behavior (e.g., overeating, vomiting)
- Analyze consequences of this behavior (cognitions, positive and negative
  reinforcers and punishments, e.g., decreased anxiety, feeling over full, losing
  or gaining weight)
- Make specific goals to modify the environment/cognitions to reduce target
  behaviors

gnitive and behavioral strategies used to promote change in diet and physical
ivity may include:

- Goal setting
- Self-monitoring
- Problem solving
- Social support
- Stress management

- Stimulus control
- Cognitive restructuring
- Relapse prevention
- Rewards/contingency management

INTERVENTION

4th Edition

Theoretical Basis/Approach (C-1)
Health Belief Model

Description
The Health Belief Model (HBM) is a psychological model that focuses on an individual's attitudes and beliefs to attempt to explain and predict health behaviors. The HBM is based on the assumption that an individual will be motivated to take health-related action if that person (1) feels that a negative health condition (e.g., diabetes) can be avoided or managed, (2) has a positive expectation that by taking a recommended action, he or she will avoid negative health consequences (e.g., good blood glucose control will preserve eye sight), and (3) believes he or she can successfully perform a recommended health action (e.g., I can use carbohydrate counting and control my diet. I can engage in regular physical activity).

Implication for Counseling Interventions
The Health Belief Model is particularly helpful to practitioners planning interventions targeted to individuals with clinical nutrition-related risk factors, such as diabetes, high blood cholesterol, and/or hypertension. The six major constructs of the model have been found to be important in impacting an individual's motivation to take health-related action. The following table provides definitions and application guidance for the key constructs of the theory. Motivational interviewing strategies may be appropriate to address perceived susceptibility, severity, benefits, and barriers. Behavioral strategies are most appropriate once the patient/client begins to take action to modify his or her diet and/or physical activity.

These six constructs are useful components in designing behavior change programs. It is important for the practitioner to understand the patient's perception of the health threat and potential benefits of treatment. According to the HBM, an asymptomatic diabetic may not be compliant with his or her treatment regiment if he or she does not:

- believe he or she has diabetes (susceptibility)
- believe diabetes will seriously impact his or her life (perceived seriousness)
- believe following the diabetic diet will decrease the negative effects of diabetes (perceived benefits)
- believe the effort to follow the diet is worth the benefit to be gained (perceived barriers)
- have stimulus to initiate action (cue to action)
- have confidence in their ability to achieve success (self-efficacy)

Updated: 2013 Edition

INTERVENTION

Theoretical Basis/Approach (C-1)

Health Belief Model

Constructs

Perceived susceptibility

Client's belief or opinion of the personal threat a health condition represents for them; client opinion regarding whether they have the condition (e.g., diabetes or hypertension) or their chance of getting the disease or condition

Strategies

- Educate on disease/condition risk factors
- Tailor information to the client
- Ask client if they think they are at risk or have the disease/condition
- Guided discussions
- Motivational interviewing (express empathy, open-ended questions, reflective listening, affirming, summarizing, and eliciting self-motivation statements)

Perceived severity

Client's belief about the impact a particular health threat will have on them and their lifestyle

Strategies

- Educate on consequences of the disease/condition; show graphs, statistics
- Elicit client response
- Discuss potential impact on client's lifestyle
- Motivational interviewing

Perceived benefits and barriers

Client's belief regarding benefits they will derive from taking nutrition-related action; perceived benefits versus barriers—client's perception of whether benefits will outweigh the sacrifices and efforts involved in behavior change

Strategies

- Clearly define benefits of nutrition therapy and physical activity
- Role models, testimonials
- Explore ambivalence and barriers
- Imagine the future
- Explore successes
- Summarize and affirm the positive

Cues to action

Internal or external triggers that motivate or stimulate action

Strategies

- How-to education
- Incentive programs
- Link current symptoms to disease/condition
- Discuss media information
- Reminder phone calls/mailings
- Social support

Self-efficacy

Client confidence in their ability to successfully accomplish the necessary action

Strategies

- Skill training/demonstration
- Introduce alternatives and choices
- Behavior contracting; small, incremental goals
- Coaching, verbal reinforcement

INTERVENTION

Theoretical Basis/Approach (C-1)
Social Learning Theory

Description

Social Learning Theory, also known as Social Cognitive Theory, provides a framework for understanding, predicting, and changing behavior. The theory identifies a dynamic, reciprocal relationship between environment, the person, and behavior. The person can be both an agent for change and a responder to change. It emphasizes the importance of observing and modeling behaviors, attitudes and emotional reactions of others. Determinants of behavior include goals, outcome expectations, and self-efficacy. Reinforcements increase or decrease the likelihood that the behavior will be repeated.

Implication for Counseling Interventions

Social Learning Theory is rich in concepts applicable to nutrition counseling. The following table provides definitions and application guidance for the key concepts of the theory.

INTERVENTION

Theoretical Basis/Approach (C-1)

Social Learning Theory

Concepts

Reciprocal Determinism

A person's ability to change a behavior is influenced by characteristics within the person (e.g., beliefs), the environment, and the behavior itself (e.g., difficulty doing the behavior). All three interact to influence if the behavior change will happen.

Strategies

Consider multiple behavior change strategies targeting motivation, action, the individual and the environment:

- Motivational interviewing
- Social support
- Skill development training/coaching
- Stimulus control
- Demonstration

Behavioral Capability

The knowledge and skills that are needed for a person to change behavior

Strategies

- Comprehensive education
- Demonstration
- Skill development training/coaching

Expectations

For a person to do a behavior, they must believe that the behavior will result in outcomes important to them

Strategies

- Motivational interviewing
- Model positive outcomes of diet/exercise

Self-Efficacy

Confidence in ability to take action and persist in action

Strategies

- Break task down to component parts
- Demonstration/modeling
- Skill development training/coaching
- Reinforcement
- Small, incremental goals/ behavioral contracting

Observational Learning

When a person learns how to do a behavior by watching credible others do the same behavior

Strategies

- Demonstrations
- Role modeling
- Group problem-solving sessions

Reinforcement

Response to a behavior that will either increase or decrease the likelihood that the behavior will be repeated

- Affirm accomplishments
- Encourage self reward/self-reinforcement
- Incentives for process components of change (e.g., keeping a food diary or physical activity log)

INTERVENTION

Theoretical Basis/Approach (C-1)

Transtheoretical Model/Stages of Change

Definition

A theoretical model of intentional health behavior change that describes a sequence of cognitive (attitudes and intentions) and behavioral steps people take in successful behavior change. The model, developed by Prochaska and DiClemente, is composed of a core concept known as Stages of Change, a series of independent variables, the Processes of Change, and outcome measures including decision balance and self-efficacy. The model has been used to guide development of effective interventions for a variety of health behaviors.

Implication for Counseling Interventions

One of the defining characteristics of this model is that it describes behavior change not as a discrete event (e.g., today I am going to stop overeating), but as something that occurs in stages, over time. The five stages reflect an individual's attitudes, intentions and behavior related to change of a specific behavior and include the following:

- Precontemplation – no recognition of need for change; no intention to take action within the next 6 months
- Contemplation – recognition of need to change; intends to take action within the next 6 months
- Preparation – intends to take action in the next 30 days and has taken some behavioral steps in that direction
- Action – has made changes in target behavior for less than 6 months
- Maintenance – has changed target behavior for more than 6 months

Determination of a patient/client stage of change is relatively simple, involving a few questions regarding intentions and current diet. One of the appealing aspects of the theory is that the Process of Change construct describes cognitive and behavioral activities or strategies, which may be applied at various stages to move a person forward through the stages of change. This movement is not always linear, and patients can cycle in and out of various stages. The model has been used to effectively tailor interventions to the needs of clients at various stages. Knowing a patient/client's stage of change can help a practitioner determine:

- Whether intervention now is appropriate
- The type and content of intervention to use (motivational versus action oriented)
- Appropriate and timely questions about past efforts, pros and cons of change, obstacles, challenges and potential strategies
- The amount of time to spend with the patient

The table on the next page provides guidance for applying stages and processes of change to the adoption of healthful diets.

This theoretical basis/approach has also been used with regard to physical activity.

Theoretical Basis/Approach (C-1)

Transtheoretical Model/Stages of Change

General guidelines for Applying Stages and Processes of Change to Adoption of Healthful Diets

State of readiness (Key strategies for moving to next stage)	Treatment do's and don'ts at this stage
Precontemplation (Increased information and awareness, emotional acceptance)	• Provide personalized information. • Allow client to express emotions about his or her disease or about the need to make dietary changes. • Do not assume the client has knowledge or expect that providing information will automatically lead to behavior change. • Do not ignore client's emotional adjustment to the need for dietary change, which could override ability to process relevant information.
Contemplation (Increased confidence in one's ability to adopt recommended behaviors)	• Discuss and resolve barriers to dietary change. • Encourage support networks. • Give positive feedback about a client's abilities. • Help to clarify ambivalence about adopting behavior and emphasize expected benefits. • Do not ignore the potential impact of family members, and others, on client's ability to comply. • Do not be alarmed by or critical of a client's ambivalence.
Preparation (Resolution of ambivalence, firm commitment, and specific action plan)	• Encourage client to set specific, achievable goals (e.g., use 1% milk instead of whole milk). • Reinforce small changes that client may have already achieved. • Do not recommend general behavior changes (e.g., "Eat less fat"). • Do not refer to small changes as "not good enough."
Action (Behavioral skill training and social support)	• Refer to education program for self-management skills. • Provide self-help materials. • Do not refer clients to information-only classes.
Maintenance (Problem-solving skills and social and environmental support)	• Encourage client to anticipate and plan for potential difficulties (e.g., maintaining dietary changes on vacation). • Collect information about local resources (e.g., support groups, shopping guides). • Encourage client to "recycle" if he or she has a lapse or relapse. • Recommend more challenging dietary changes if client is motivated. • Do not assume that initial action means permanent change. • Do not be discouraged or judgmental about a lapse or relapse.

Source: Adapted from Kristal AR, Glanz K, Curry S, Patterson RE. How can stages of change be best used in dietary interventions? *J Am Diet Assoc*. 1999;99:683.

Prochaska recommends the following strategies, which target motivation, be used in the early stages of change: consciousness raising, dramatic relief (e.g., emotional arousal via role playing or personal testimonials), environmental reevaluation (e.g., empathy training and family interactions), social liberation (e.g., advocacy, empowerment) and self-reevaluation (e.g., value clarification, healthy role models and imagery). These strategies are very consistent with motivational interviewing techniques. In the later stages of change, behavioral strategies are most appropriate.

INTERVENTION

Strategies (C-2)

Definition
An evidence-based method or plan of action designed to achieve a particular goal. Application of behavior change theories in nutrition practice has provided practitioners with a collection of evidence-based strategies to promote behavior change. Some strategies target change in motivation and intention to change, and others target behavior change. Food and nutrition professionals selectively apply strategies based on patient/client goals and objectives, and their personal counseling philosophy and skill.

Application Guidance
An intervention typically incorporates tools and strategies derived from a variety of behavior change theories and models. The practitioner is asked to indicate which Strategies (C-2) he or she used in a particular intervention session along with the Theories (C-1) that most influence the intervention being documented.

Details of Intervention
A typical intervention might be further described with the following details. RDs/food and nutrition professionals recommend, implement, or order nutrition interventions and the action(s) may be to initiate, modify or discontinue a nutrition intervention(s):

The following strategies have proven valuable in providing effective nutrition-related (e.g. nutrition therapy, physical activity) behavior change.

- Motivational interviewing
- Goal setting
- Self-monitoring
- Problem solving
- Social support
- Stress management
- Stimulus control
- Cognitive restructuring
- Relapse prevention
- Rewards/contingency management
- Other

Additional information regarding each of the above strategies can be found within this reference sheet.

See reference manual for list of nutrition diagnoses, etiologies and signs and symptoms that often are associated with this intervention.

Strategies (C-2)

Other considerations (e.g., patient/client negotiation, patient/client needs and desires, and readiness to change)

- Lifestyle factors
- Language barrier
- Educational level
- Culture
- Socioeconomic status

Updated: Edition 2013

INTERVENTION

Strategies (C-2)

Strategy descriptions and application guidance

Motivational interviewing (MI)

A directive, client-centered counseling style for eliciting behavior change by helping clients to explore and resolve ambivalence. The approach involves selective responses to client speech in a way that helps the client resolve ambivalence and move toward change. The four guiding principles that underlie this counseling approach include:

- Express empathy
- Roll with resistance
- Develop discrepancy
- Support self-efficacy

The following specific practitioner behaviors are characteristic of the MI style:

- Expressing acceptance and affirmation
- Eliciting and selectively reinforcing the client's own self motivational statements, expressions of problem recognition, concern, desire, intention to change and ability to change
- Monitoring the client's degree of readiness to change, and ensuring that jumping ahead of the client does not generate resistance
- Affirming the client's freedom of choice and self-direction

The source of motivation is presumed to reside within the client and the counselor encourages the client to explore ambivalence, motivation and possibilities to change, so it is the client who chooses what to change, determines the change plan and strategy.

MI is an evidence-based counseling strategy which builds on Carl Roger's client centered counseling model, Prochaska and DiClemente's transtheoretical model of change, Milton Rokeach's human values theory and Daryl Bern's theory of self perception.

Implementation Tips

Tone of counseling:

- Partnership
- Nonjudgmental
- Empathetic/supportive/encouraging
- Nonconfrontational
- Quiet and eliciting

The client does most of the talking and the counselor guides the client to explore and resolve ambivalence by:

- Asking open ended questions
- Listening reflectively
- Summarizing
- Affirming
- Eliciting self-motivational statements
- Shared agenda setting/decision making
- Allowing clients to interpret information
- Rolling with resistance, rather than confronting
- Building discrepancy
- Eliciting "change talk"
- Negotiating a change plan

Strategies (C-2)

Motivational interviewing is best applied in situations when a patient is not ready, is unwilling or ambivalent about changing their diet or lifestyle.

MI integrates well with the readiness to change model to move individuals from the early stages to the action stage of change.

MI is a major paradigm change from the problem solving oriented counseling frequently employed by practitioners.

MI is not a set of techniques that can be learned quickly, but a style or approach to counseling.

Goal setting

A collaborative activity between the client and the practitioner in which the client decides from all potential activity recommendations what changes he/she will expend effort to implement.

Implementation Tips

- Appropriate for patients ready to make dietary and physical activity changes
- Coach on goal setting skills
- Document and track progress toward short-term and long-term goals
- Probe client about pros and cons of proposed goals
- Assist client in gaining the knowledge and skills necessary to succeed
- Encourage strategies to build confidence (discuss realistic steps and start with easily achievable goals)
- Aid clients in building a supportive environment
- Celebrate successes

Self-monitoring

A technique that involves keeping a detailed record of behaviors that influence diet and/or weight and may include:

- What, when, how much eaten
- Activities during eating
- Emotions and cognitions related to meals/snacks
- Frequency, duration and intensity of exercise
- Target nutrient content of foods consumed (i.e., calories/kcal/kJ, fat, fiber)
- Event, thoughts about event, emotional response, behavioral response
- Negative self-talk, replacement thoughts
- Blood glucose, blood pressure

Self-monitoring is associated with improved treatment outcomes.

Implementation Tips

- Provide rationale and instructions for self-monitoring
- Review and identify patterns
- Assist with problem solving and goal setting
- Celebrate successes
- The amount of feedback required typically diminishes as patient/client skill improves

INTERVENTION

Strategies (C-2)

Problem solving

Techniques that are taught to assist clients in identifying barriers to achieving goals, identifying and implementing solutions and evaluating the effectiveness of the solutions.

Implementation Tips

Work collaboratively with client to:

- Define the problem
- Brainstorm solutions
- Weigh pros/cons of potential solutions
- Select/implement strategy
- Evaluate outcomes
- Adjust strategy

Social support

Increased availability of social support for dietary and physical activity behavior change. Social support may be generated among an individual's family, church, school, co-workers, health club or community.

Implementation Tips

A dietetics practitioner may assist a client by:

- Establishing a collaborative relationship
- Identifying family/community support
- Assisting clients in developing assertiveness skills.
- Utilize modeling, skill training, respondent and operant conditioning
- Conducting education in a group
- Encourage family involvement

Stress management

Reaction to stress can cause some clients to loss their appetite and others to overeat. Dietetics practitioners are particularly interested in management of stressful situations, which result in less-than-optimal eating behaviors.

Implementation Tips

Two approaches may be used to manage stress, one focuses on changing the environment, and the other focuses on modifying the client's response to stress.

Environmental-focused strategies may include:

- Guidance on planning ahead
- Use of time-management skills
- Developing a support system
- Building skills to prepare quick and healthful meals, incorportate exercise
- Guidance on eating on the run

Emotion-focused strategies may include:

- Use of positive self-talk
- Building assertiveness in expressing eating desires
- Setting realistic goals
- Learning to deal appropriately with emotion-driven eating cravings
- Relaxation exercises

Strategies (C-2)

Stimulus control

Identifying and modifying social or environmental cues or triggers to act, which encourage undesirable behaviors relevant to diet and exercise. In accordance with operant conditioning principles, attention is given to reinforcement and rewards.

Implementation Tips

Review of self-monitoring records with clients may help to identify triggers for undesirable eating

Assist client in identifying ways to modify the environment to eliminate triggers. This may include things such as:

- Keeping food out of sight
- Removing high sugar/high fat snacks from the house
- Bringing lunch to work
- Establishing a rule – no eating in the car
- Help client establish criteria for rewards for desirable behavior
- Ensure reward (reinforcement) received only if criteria met

Cognitive restructuring

Techniques used to increase client awareness of their perceptions of themselves and their beliefs related to diet, weight and weight loss expectations.

Implementation Tips

Self-monitoring and techniques such as the ABC Technique of Irrational Beliefs may help clients to become more aware of thoughts that interfere in their ability to meet behavioral goals

Help clients replace dysfunctional thoughts with more rationale ones:

- Challenge shoulds, oughts, musts
- Decatastrophize expected outcomes
- Confront faulty self-perceptions
- Decenter by envisioning other perspectives

Coach clients on replacing negative self-talk with more positive, empowering and affirming statements

Relapse prevention

Techniques used to help clients prepare to address high-risk situations for relapse with appropriate strategies and thinking. Incorporates both cognitive and behavioral strategies to enhance long-term behavior change outcomes.

Implementation Tips

Assist clients:

- Assess if external circumstances are contributing to lapse, e.g., loss of job or support system
- Identify high-risk situations for slips
- Analyze reactions to slips
- Acquire knowledge and skills necessary to address high-risk situations
- Gain confidence in their ability to succeed in high-risk situations

INTERVENTION

Strategies (C-2)

Rewards/contingency management

A systematic process by which behaviors can be changed through the use of reward for specific actions. Rewards may be derived from the client or the provider.

Implementation Tips

- Provide rewards for desired behaviors, e.g., attendance, diet progress, consistent self-monitoring, physical activity
- Rewards can be monetary, prizes, parking space, gift certificates
- Assist clients in determining rewards for achievement
- Ensure rewards are not received if progress is not made

Collaboration and Referral of Nutrition Care (RC-1)

Definition

Facilitating services or interventions with other professionals, institutions, or agencies on behalf of the patient/client prior to discharge from nutrition care.

Details of Intervention

A typical intervention might be further described with the following details. RDs/food and nutrition professionals recommend, implement, or order nutrition interventions and the action(s) may be to initiate, modify or discontinue a nutrition intervention(s):

- Team meeting (Holding a team meeting to develop a comprehensive plan of care)
- Referral to RD/nutrition professional with different expertise (A referral for care by other food and nutrition professionals who provide different expertise)
- Collaborate with other nutrition professionals (Collaboration by nutrition professional with other nutrition professionals)
- Collaborate with other providers (Collaboration with others such as the physician, dentist, physical therapist, social worker, occupational therapist, speech therapist, nurse, pharmacist, or other specialist dietitian)
- Referral to other provider (Refer to others such as the physician, dentist, physical therapist, social worker, occupational therapist, speech therapist, nurse, pharmacist, or other specialist dietitian/nutrition professional)
- Referral to community agencies/programs (Refer to an appropriate agency/program (e.g., home delivered meals), assistance programs for women, infants and children (e.g.WIC), food assistance programs (e.g., food pantry, soup kitchen, food stamps) housing assistance, shelters, rehabilitation, physical and mental disability programs, education training, and employment programs))

See reference manual for list of nutrition diagnoses, etiologies and signs and symptoms that often are associated with this intervention.

Other considerations (e.g., patient/client negotiation, patient/client needs and desires, and readiness to change)

- Availability of services related to patient/client need (specialty dietitians, clinical pharmacists, speech pathologists, nurse practitioners, etc.)
- Anticipated duration of health care encounter/hospital or long-term care discharge
- Resources available for care
- Government medical programs (e.g., Medicare/Medicaid) insurance guidelines and restrictions
- Food assistance program (e.g., food stamp program) guidelines and regulations

Updated: 2013 Edition

INTERVENTION

Discharge and Transfer of Nutrition Care to a New Setting or Provider (RC-2)

Definition
Discharge planning and transfer of nutrition care from one level or location of care to another.

Details of Intervention
A typical intervention might be further described with the following details. Food and nutrition professionals recommend, implement, or order nutrition interventions and the action(s) may be to initiate, modify or discontinue a nutrition intervention(s

- Discharge and transfer to other providers: Refer to others such as the physician, dentist, physical therapist, social worker, occupational therapist, speech therapist, nurse, or pharmacist
- Discharge and transfer to community agencies/programs: Refer to a community agency/program (e.g., home delivered meals, assistance programs for women, infants and children [e.g.,WIC], food assistance programs [e.g., food pantry, soup kitchen, food stamps], housing assistance, shelters, rehabilitation physical and mental disability programs, education, training and employment programs)
- Discharge and transfer to another nutrition professional: Transfer of nutrition care to another food and nutrition professional

See reference manual for list of nutrition diagnoses, etiologies and signs and symptor that often are associated with this intervention.

Other considerations (e.g., patient/client negotiation, patient/client needs and desires, and readiness to change)

- Availability of discharge planning services, options for care
- Preferences for the level and location of care
- Resources available for care
- Government medical programs (e.g. Medicare/Medicaid), insurance guidelines and restrictions
- Health literacy
- Ability to implement treatment at home
- Food assistance program (e.g., food stamp program) guidelines and regulations

Updated: 2013 Edition

SNAPshot
NCP Step 4. Nutrition Monitoring and Evaluation

What is the purpose of nutrition monitoring and evaluation? The purpose is to determine the amount of progress made and whether goals/expected outcomes are being met. Nutrition monitoring and evaluation identifies patient/client* outcomes relevant to the nutrition diagnosis and intervention plans and goals. Nutrition care outcomes—the desired results of nutrition care—are defined in this step. The change in specific nutrition care indicators between assessment and reassessment can be measured and compared to the patient/client's previous status, nutrition intervention goals, or reference standards. The aim is to promote more uniformity within the dietetics profession in assessing the effectiveness of nutrition intervention.

How does a food and nutrition professional determine what to measure for nutrition monitoring and evaluation? Practitioners select nutrition care indicators that will reflect a change as a result of nutrition care. In addition, food and nutrition professionals will consider factors such as the nutrition diagnosis and its etiology and signs or symptoms, the nutrition intervention, medical diagnosis, health care outcome goals, quality management goals for nutrition, practice setting, patient/client population, and disease state and/or severity.

How are outcomes used in nutrition monitoring and evaluation organized? In four categories**:

Food/Nutrition-Related History Outcomes—*Food and nutrient intake, food and nutrient administration, medication/herbal supplement use, knowledge/beliefs, food and supplies availability, physical activity, nutrition quality of life*

Anthropometric Measurement Outcomes—*Height, weight, body mass index (BMI), growth pattern indices/percentile ranks, and weight history*

Biochemical Data, Medical Tests, and Procedure Outcomes—*Lab data (e.g., electrolytes, glucose) and tests (e.g., gastric emptying time, resting metabolic rate)*

Nutrition-Focused Physical Finding Outcomes—*Physical appearance, muscle and fat wasting, swallow function, appetite, and affect*

*patient/client refers to individuals, groups, populations, family members, and/or caregivers.

**While the domains, classes, and terms for nutrition assessment and nutrition monitoring and evaluation combined, there are no nutrition care outcomes associated with the domain entitled Client History. Terms from this domain are used for nutrition assessment only and do not change as a result of nutrition intervention.

MONITOR & EVAL

What does nutrition monitoring and evaluation involve? Practitioners do three thin[g]s as part of nutrition monitoring and evaluation—monitor, measure, and evaluate t[he] changes in nutrition care indicators—to determine patient/client progress. Practitione[rs] monitor by providing evidence that the nutrition intervention is or is not changing t[he] patient/client's behavior or status. They measure outcomes by collecting data on t[he] appropriate nutrition outcome indicator(s). Finally, food and nutrition profession[als] compare the current findings with previous status, nutrition intervention goals, an[d/] or reference standards (i.e., criteria) and evaluate the overall impact of the nutriti[on] intervention on the patient/client's health outcomes. The use of standardized indicat[or] and criteria increases the validity and reliability in how outcome data are collected. [All] these procedures facilitate electronic charting, coding, and outcomes measurement.

> **Critical thinking during this step…**
> - Selecting appropriate indicators/measures
> - Using appropriate reference standards for comparison
> - Defining where patient/client is in terms of expected outcomes
> - Explaining a variance from expected outcomes
> - Determining factors that help or hinder progress
> - Deciding between discharge and continuation of nutrition care

Are food and nutrition professionals limited to the nutrition monitoring and evaluation outcomes terms? A cascade of outcomes of nutrition care have been identified; each outcome has several possible indicators that can be measured depending on the patient/client population, practice setting, and disease state/ severity. Food and nutrition professionals can propose additions or revisions using the Procedure for Nutrition Controlled Vocabulary/Terminology Maintenance/Revi[ew] available from the Academy.

Detailed information about this step can be found in the Academy of Nutrition and Dietetics' Internationa[l] Dietetics and Nutrition Terminology (IDNT) Reference Manual: Standardized Language for the Nutrition Care Process, Fourth Edition.

Terminology Index